Trauma Informed Care

I0035003

This practical guide introduces and critically examines the concept of trauma informed care, exploring how it can be implemented in everyday nursing and midwifery practice across a range of settings. Supporting nurses and midwives to integrate trauma informed knowledge and practice into their work, this comprehensive book begins with an overview of what trauma means. It looks at theories of trauma and the neuroscience of trauma and memory. It discusses the diagnostics of trauma and considers how trauma impacts relationships (including those within healthcare settings), and health, illness, and recovery. It also investigates how trauma can affect people differently across the lifespan and contexts.

The second part of the book builds on the first, focusing on how an understanding of trauma can inform nursing and midwifery practice across settings. It looks at promoting safety in interpersonal relationships, navigating interventions, talking about trauma, responding after potentially traumatic events, and responding to trauma, self-care, and systemic challenges. This book provides essential knowledge around trauma informed care relevant to nurses and midwives, and uses a range of approaches to help readers transfer learning to their own practice.

It is an essential guide for nurses and midwives in practice and in training across the full range of practice settings.

Sophie Isobel is an Associate Professor in the School of Nursing, Faculty of Medicine and Health at the University of Sydney, Australia.

Trauma Informed Care

A Guide for Nursing and Midwifery Practice

Sophie Isobel

Routledge
Taylor & Francis Group

LONDON AND NEW YORK

Designed cover image: Sophie Isobel

First published 2026
by Routledge
4 Park Square, Milton Park, Abingdon, Oxon OX14 4RN

and by Routledge
605 Third Avenue, New York, NY 10158

Routledge is an imprint of the Taylor & Francis Group, an informa business

For Product Safety Concerns and Information please contact our EU
representative GPSR@taylorandfrancis.com. Taylor & Francis Verlag
GmbH, Kaufingerstraße 24, 80331 München, Germany.

Trademark notice: Product or corporate names may be trademarks or
registered trademarks, and are used only for identification and explanation
without intent to infringe.

British Library Cataloguing-in-Publication Data
A catalogue record for this book is available from the British Library

ISBN: 978-1-032-87066-3 (hbk)
ISBN: 978-1-032-87052-6 (pbk)
ISBN: 978-1-003-53077-0 (ebk)

DOI: 10.4324/9781003530770

Typeset in Bembo
by KnowledgeWorks Global Ltd.

Contents

Preface

This book tries to be trauma informed. As such, it is important to start with an overview of what it includes. This is not a trigger warning because it is not possible for me to know how other people may experience these stories and ideas, but it is a content preface. This book talks directly about trauma. It uses examples of trauma, of shame, of good practice, of less good practice, and of complexity. It doesn't include details about experiences, events, or situations that aren't needed; mostly, details aren't needed. But it does try to shine a light on trauma, which involves acknowledging it, exploring it, imagining it, and considering it. It is based on an understanding that trauma impacts many people's lives and that there are things we can do as nurses and midwives to try to be sensitive to this in the context of care.

This book is a gathering of work and thoughts developed over many years. In that time, I have worked with many people. Most examples are a mash-up of various experiences and people in one. The examples used in this book are adapted from real things, many from clients but also from friends, family, and my own life. I have adapted them where needed to ensure privacy. Thus, nothing was perhaps quite as it is written, but also nothing important is made up.

In my nursing career, I think I was always aware of trauma, but I didn't always have the words to describe it. There were parts of my work that I found hard, things that had to be done to people that felt intrusive, people who seemed to react in unexpected ways to the provision of care, and ways that I was personally changed by my nursing work and experiences. I have worked most of my nursing career in mental health settings, but I am also an early childhood nurse, and I have worked a lot with children, families, and infants. I have worked most of my career trying to improve the experiences of care for people and their families, in various ways. In 2012, when I was working in a large metropolitan mental health service, I led a practice development project to help support the nurses on an acute inpatient unit with their practice. It was a time of high acuity in services and a lack of staff and resources. That is, a time in mental health services that was much like any other time. I had never heard of Trauma Informed Care. But to start the project, the project team and I listened to what the nurses were struggling with in their roles. The nurses described not being sure how to help people who were repeatedly presenting and didn't seem to benefit from care, people who were aggressive towards staff, and people who engaged in sustained or repeated self-harm. We considered tackling each of these in turn, but instead we took a different approach and focused on what may underpin these experiences. In engaging with the work coming out of the United States at the time, the project became 'trauma informed care'.

That small practice development project changed the course of my career. It changed the way I think about nursing, it gave me language to talk about the work, and it led me to engage with nurses and clinicians across settings and across the world. It also changed how I understood my own life and that of my family. It changed how I interact in life and how I move through the world. I have learnt that trauma informed ways of being are not just relevant to mental health care; they are relevant to all human services and have particular importance across all parts of nursing and midwifery. I haven't yet found a part of nursing and midwifery where they aren't relevant.

My understanding of what it means to be informed in my ways of being, by trauma, is a commitment to ongoing learning, reflection, and listening. This means that this book cannot be a handbook of 'how to be a trauma informed nurse or midwife'. Knowledge will develop and change; hopefully, social and political responses to trauma will develop and change, and how trauma affects people will also always develop and change. Language about trauma will likely change too. In the time I have been writing this book, the world has been recovering from a global pandemic, weather patterns have been extreme and dramatic, and wars have broken out and continued. Alongside these events, people have also continued to experience trauma within their homes, relationships, families, and lives. Understandings of trauma are constantly evolving, and as such, this book is a guide for how to begin to think about trauma, and a reflection on some of the ways that knowledge of trauma generally can inform our practice as nurses and midwives, but there may be bits that don't fit with everyone's understanding.

I started off writing this book in a usual textbook way, without my own voice and thoughts included. But at some point, they snuck in. All of the knowledge and experiences from my own life, as a nurse, as a parent, as a child, as a trauma survivor, as a therapist, as a human, have helped me learn how to be trauma informed. This book isn't about me, and it doesn't include any unnecessary details about any of these parts of my life, but it is also about me. It is about any of us who have experienced trauma or who provide care to those who have. In the end, I didn't want to write it as though I am not here, saying the words, making sense of it, drawing on things that have really happened, and making sense of them in evolving ways as best I can. Trauma is a dehumanising experience. It tells us that we are insignificant or not worthwhile. It teaches us ways to blame ourselves, shame ourselves, and hide ourselves. It makes us feel shame for the actions of others. Thus, to be trauma informed is to resist the communal, social, and individual shaming and silencing that enables trauma. This isn't easy. It is not a state; it is a daily practice. But I strive daily to not be complicit in trauma sustaining ways of being anymore. With this in mind, I wrote this book in the best way that I could.

Engaging with trauma is not easy. It will always be uncomfortable, lest we become complacent. I have come to see that working in the space of trauma requires unapologetic commitments to radical forms of self-care. I spent the last stages of writing this book in a peaceful forest, caring for my soul and mind as part of the work of going over and over these words about trauma. This is a privilege and extreme act of self-care, but part of the work of nursing and midwifery will always be about sustaining ourselves as we go about caring for others. And part of being trauma informed in nursing and midwifery involves looking after ourselves as we hold the trauma of others. While escaping to a forest is not always possible, do what you need to do to look after yourself as you read this text.

Acknowledgements

Acknowledging people living with trauma

People who have experienced trauma may varyingly identify as victims or survivors or may prefer to not identify with what has happened to them in their past at all. In this book, the phrase 'people who have experienced trauma' is mostly used, with acknowledgment that for some people the trauma is ongoing, and there may also be others who do not frame their experiences as trauma.

Trauma is widespread. It impacts people of all genders, classes, sexualities, races, ages, and demographics. While at a population level it may impact some groups disproportionately, it is not possible to say that someone's experience of overwhelming fear, betrayal, horror, or loss of self is less significant than someone else's. People who have experienced, or are experiencing trauma, are not a small group in society, although they remain largely hidden. There are people in every room who have experienced trauma. This book is written in acknowledgement of all those people in every room.

Trauma, as this book will explore, arises from a great many human experiences and impacts people in varying ways. Some people get through life with less apparent impacts, while for others, the shadow of trauma is ever-present. In talking about 'trauma' and delivering care to 'people who have experienced trauma', we should never forget that this could be any of us or people we love. However, while many of us have experienced trauma, this does not mean we know what it is to be someone else who has experienced trauma. I cannot speak for anyone else about their experience of trauma, and no healthcare worker should ever presume they know exactly what any other human needs in the aftermath of trauma. People who have survived or are surviving trauma are not a homogeneous group and nor should they be assumed to be. I acknowledge that trauma is messy and people's stories and ways of expressing trauma may also be.

Acknowledging imperfect language

I recognise that trauma will impact the lives, families, and communities of nurses and midwives who may be reading this book. At times, the words used or the descriptions given may not resonate with you. Language also changes over time, and while I have tried to use inclusive words and phrases, I recognise (and hope) that language around trauma will continue to evolve to become more sensitive and refined. Where needed, key terms are defined in this context but, of course, no term is perfect, and experiences of trauma are diverse and can be difficult to classify or categorise. I also use a lot of metaphoric descriptions, which may not be usual in a nursing textbook. Yet metaphors exist to help us try to understand things which are difficult to understand. Trauma is not an exact thing; it is a felt experience, and it is different for everyone. Similarly, trauma informed care is largely about how care feels. It is important in trying to understand trauma and trauma informed care that we have ways of imagining how things feel, even if we haven't felt them ourselves. I find that metaphoric language helps anchor unknown things to known things, thereby making the incomprehensible somewhat comprehensible.

Acknowledging cultural trauma on the land where this book was written

In Australia, where I wrote this book, it is not possible to write about trauma and not recognise the historical and ongoing trauma inflicted on First Nations communities. Aboriginal people in Australia and across the world have endured trauma across generations and have in-depth knowledge of the loss and pain of trauma, as well as ways of surviving and healing. I also acknowledge that I wrote this book guided by a worldview heavily influenced by colonial understandings of 'trauma' and in line with the practices of mainstream health services where many Aboriginal people continue to experience structural and systemic violence.

   I wrote this book on the unceded land of the Gadigal people in Sydney, Australia, where I am lucky to live, work, and walk. It always was and always will be Aboriginal land.

Introduction

It is essential that a large part of this book focuses on trauma. Sometimes people want to get the brief overview of trauma and move quickly on to 'what does it mean in practice to be trauma informed'. Especially as nurses and midwives, there is so little time to spend within work hours on engaging with ideas and deep thinking. I understand the need to ensure concepts translate into practical and tangible actions. The second half of this book will focus on what trauma informed care means in practice, and I have tried to be as specific and practice oriented as possible. However, there is a risk in focusing just on what 'trauma informed care' means, without attempting to really engage with the details of trauma. We need to understand trauma for care to be informed by it. We need to understand it in enough depth that we can be flexible and sensitive in how we use that knowledge to inform our care. Therefore, the first half of this book is about what trauma is, and the second part explores how you can begin to use this knowledge to inform nursing and midwifery practice. It has been my experience that if enough time is spent on understanding trauma, then what it means to be trauma informed flows almost unavoidably from this. Once you start to think about, recognise, and be curious about trauma, practice and interactions look and feel different. It is this that is trauma informed care. So, it is necessary to begin with trauma.

Introducing trauma

Experiences of trauma are not uncommon, and knowledge of trauma is not new. The word trauma has different meanings in different contexts, including within nursing and midwifery. In the context of this book, it refers to the lasting impacts of experiences which are overwhelming, scary, distressing, or harmful.

> Trauma in the context of this book refers to the lasting impacts of experiences which are overwhelming, scary, distressing, or harmful.

Like other words which describe human experiences like 'love' or 'pain', diverse and differing experiences are covered by the one term. 'Trauma' is used to describe physical injuries and scars, life-changing events, experiences of distress, disorders and symptom clusters, pervasive ways of seeing the world, and patterns of dysregulation. It includes

DOI: 10.4324/9781003530770-1

things or moments which shock or horrify us, and it includes pervasive experiences that impact us in ongoing ways.

Judith Herman describes:

> Psychological trauma is an affiliation of the powerless. At the moment of trauma, the victim is rendered helpless by overwhelming force. When the force is that of nature, we speak of disasters. When the force is that of other human beings, we speak of atrocities. Traumatic events overwhelm the ordinary systems of care that give people a sense of control, connection, and meaning … Traumatic events are extraordinary, not because they occur rarely, but rather because they overwhelm the ordinary human adaptations to life. Unlike commonplace misfortunes, traumatic events generally involve threats to life or bodily integrity, or a close personal encounter with violence and death. They confront human beings with the extremities of helplessness and terror and evoke the responses of catastrophe.
>
> (Herman, 1992, p. 33)

Writing about trauma is challenging. Finding a definition that doesn't exclude or overly include is also challenging. There are disagreements about what trauma is, there are sensitivities in ensuring types of trauma are included, there are issues of power and privilege inherent in knowledge production and dissemination, and there are differing preferences for how to refer to people who have experienced trauma. While there is a constant emerging understanding of the ways that trauma can impact the brain, health, illness, recovery, and life, and increasing discourse around trauma in the lives of people, trauma has always existed. People who are admitted to hospital, people receiving care in the community, people having babies, people who are sick, people who are dying, may all have experiences of trauma that may or may not be relevant to the care they are currently receiving. Partners, family members, and friends of people receiving care may have experienced trauma. And, of course, healthcare professionals, doctors, nurses, and others too may have trauma. This book exists because trauma exists and is common, and this book exists because there are things that can be done to make experiences of giving and receiving healthcare less likely to cause trauma, activate past experiences of trauma, or compound trauma. While formal ideas of being 'trauma informed' have emerged in the last 30 years or so, whether it has been called 'trauma informed care' or not, there has been knowledge and wisdom related to trauma informed ways of being that have existed for much longer.

While trauma overwhelms us, it can also do so slowly, or we can develop incredible ways to cope that make it seem acceptable and manageable. The overwhelm can be overt or much more subtle. In the 1920s, Freud described trauma as something that 'breaches the protective shield around the mind' (Freud, 1922). While perhaps too metaphoric for some, and some of Freud's understandings and interpretations of trauma were certainly questionable, this description speaks to the 'wound' of psychological trauma and the disruption to assumptions of safety experienced by so many. I like this description, and I think of it often.

Building on existing and long-standing knowledge of trauma, in this book, 'trauma' refers to *the sustained effects of life-impacting experiences*. This commonly includes experiences of horror, fear, or betrayal, but can also include misuses of power or structural disadvantage or control. The term 'trauma' is also inclusive of experiences not linked to events, such as intergenerational trauma or vicarious trauma. Wherever possible, explanations are given around the differences and similarities between types of trauma, with acknowledgement that people's individual experiences are different and no explanation can ever be perfect.

Trauma is relative to context. This means that what may be horrifying and over-whelm coping capacity for one person may be vastly different from that of another, based on environment, experiences, and resources. One person's trauma may be another person's everyday world. In some countries, we turn on the TV and feel horrified by what we see, while others live their whole lives in these places. It is not possible to com-pare trauma as it is always relative to the context in which it occurs.

Trauma has disproportionately impacted some groups and communities in society. For example, Indigenous and First Nations communities around the world have histor-ically experienced significant trauma through colonisation and continue to experience structural and social disadvantage; communities of people who have survived wars or continue to experience wars have disproportionate experiences of trauma, with those living in places where resources are limited are further impacted; across the globe, women have been more likely to experience domestic traumas such as intimate partner violence or sexual abuse; and people with disabilities are more vulnerable to trauma in relationships and care. Children and young people are another group who are vulnera-ble to trauma and disproportionately impacted by its effects, whose voices are not always included in discussions about trauma. Older people's experiences may also be silenced.

Trauma informed approaches have emerged from research into trauma and move-ments led by people who have experienced trauma. They are social movements rather than discrete changes, and as such they represent the cumulative and collective efforts of people across settings. Trauma informed care emerged out of awareness of the impacts of war upon returned soldiers in the 1960s and 1970s, at a time when awareness of domestic trauma and violence was also being voiced by feminist movements. These shifts in awareness of trauma and its impacts were also aligned to activism by consumer/survivor/ex-patient movements in the 1980s where people who had experienced psychi-atric treatment were speaking out against coercion and harm in care. In the 1990s, the Adverse Childhood Experiences study started collecting and reporting large amounts of data on the implications of trauma for health across the lifespan, and concurrently the Substance Abuse and Mental Health Services Association (SAMHSA) in the United States of America began recognising and writing about the relevance of trauma to care. Fallot and Harris (Harris & Fallot, 2001) are often credited with first articulating the difference between trauma treatment services and 'trauma informed care'. Trauma informed approaches were initially heavily focused on mental health services, behav-ioural health services, and violence and trauma specific services, but they have now been taken up across sectors and services. They are now referenced within policy, practice, and service models across education, health, social services, and more. As knowledge of how trauma impacts health, well-being, and care is refined and trauma informed care articulated, it is important to recognise the building of knowledge over time. Knowledge of trauma has long existed, and many services have been working with communities who have experienced trauma, in ways that foster safety and trust, long before the phrase 'trauma informed care' was coined.

This book takes a critical lens to trauma informed approaches, seeking to ensure they are used and implemented in ways that are informed by the knowledge held by those who have experiences of trauma, including in healthcare contexts. Yet it is also under-pinned by the assumption that providing trauma informed care is essential, beneficial, and feasible. Nurses and midwives are in powerful positions to provide trauma informed care due to the nature of their relationships with people across the lifespan. Thus, this book aims to support nurses and midwives to be able to provide care and continue to undertake their challenging roles in ways that minimise harm and promote healing.

References

Freud, S. (1922). *Beyond the pleasure principle.* (E. Jones, Ed.; C. J. M. Hubback, Trans.). The International Psycho-Analytical Press. https://doi.org/10.1037/11189-000

Harris, M., & Fallot, R. D. (2001). Envisioning a trauma-informed service system: A vital paradigm shift. *New Directions for Mental Health Services, 2001*(89), 3–22. https://doi.org/10.1002/yd.23320018903

Herman, J. (1992). *Trauma and recovery.* Basic Books/Hachette Book Group.

Part I
The Theory

1 What is trauma?

Often, as nurses and midwives, we don't receive formal education around trauma. Instead, we have a sense of what it means based on our work, our personal lives, our observations, our communities, and our professional development. To be trauma informed requires understanding of what trauma is, how it impacts people and their lives, and what causes trauma. It also requires consideration of how and why trauma is relevant to healthcare. This knowledge is then used to 'inform' care.

There isn't one definition of trauma; it can mean different things to different people in different contexts. Trauma, in the context of this book, refers to the lasting psychological impacts of experiences which are overwhelming, scary, distressing, or harmful. Within this are experiences of helplessness and misuses of power and often inescapable events.

The word trauma has its roots in 17th century Greek where it referred to a wound: the physical injury left by exposure to harm. Many nurses and midwives are familiar with physical wounds from working in hospitals, emergency, acute care, rehabilitation, or maternity settings. Psychological trauma is also a wound. After any injury, there are different kinds of wounds: there are wounds that are bad, but heal fast and leave no mark; there are wounds that heal but leave permanent scars; there are wounds that are hard to heal or never quite heal; wounds which get complicated by other factors that impede healing; or wounds that we think are healed and then we move in a certain way and they suddenly open back up. This is very similar to the psychological effects of exposure to harm. Some things hurt us badly for a short period and then we recover. Some things change us in ways that we are never quite the same. And some things stay hurting us in the present, long after the event.

To find a definition of trauma that 'feels' right is difficult. Any definition requires suitable depth and breadth to capture the variety of things which can be traumatic, while also protecting space for the complexity and horror of many traumatic experiences. Definitions should be sufficiently flexible to allow for the differing explanatory frames that people have for the links between events and experiences, while also being structured enough to not allow any distressing thing to be classified as traumatic. They should allow scope to recognise the significant and at times predictable impact that exposure to traumatic events can have upon individuals (to inform prevention), without assuming that all adversities are experienced in the same way.

Often the definition is used where trauma refers to an event, a series of events, or a set of circumstances that is experienced by an individual as physically or emotionally harmful or life threatening and that has lasting adverse effects on the individual's functioning and mental, physical, social, emotional, or spiritual well-being (SAMHSA, 2014, p. 7). There are three components within this definition: the event, the experience, and the

DOI: 10.4324/9781003530770-3

effect. Events may be seen as traumatic; individuals may have different experiences within events or circumstances; and there may or may not be lasting traumatic effects. I have found this three-part approach helpful for thinking through trauma as a process.

Potentially traumatic events lead to trauma

Events which can be potentially traumatic usually involve fear, betrayal, helplessness, or horror, but they can also involve neglect or loss or any other overwhelming experience. Overwhelming doesn't mean that we can't cope, but that our usual coping systems are strained or ineffective. Sometimes new ways of coping are required, and these may form part of the trauma impact. There is increasing recognition that trauma can also occur from events that may not be assumed to be traumatic. For example, some young people's experiences in educational systems may be cumulatively traumatic due to feelings of inadequacy, shame, control, or bullying, while other young people thrive or enjoy schooling. In this way, the potentially traumatic event is much more woven into the experience than the event itself.

At times, the word trauma is used to refer only to the event, but it is not the event itself which is the trauma. Events can be precipitants or indicators of possible trauma, but trauma is the legacy. As understanding of trauma evolves, the concept of trauma is less linked to specific events and more understood to refer to experiences and effects. It is also recognised that people experience events differently and they may be more or less able to cope or recover.

Box 1.1: How events are experienced

If an armed robbery occurs in a bank, how everyone in the bank experiences the event will be influenced by a variety of factors and this will impact the lasting effects (or how traumatic the event is). The factors may include internal factors related to each person, for example, how old they are, what beliefs they hold about world and why things happen, whether they have experienced similar levels of fear previously, whether they have existing assumptions that the world and people are safe, as well as factors related to their context, for example, whether they have a safe place to go afterwards and supportive relationships, access to resources to engage supports, whether they have time and space to process the events, what other stressors or dangers they are facing, as well as circumstantial factors to do with the event itself, for example, how close they were standing to the robber, whether they were on their own or with someone they could trust, if they did something brave or revered, if they hid or panicked, whether they felt proud of their automatic responses in the moment, whether they got hurt, if they saw someone else get hurt … and so on. Every person in the bank will experience the robbery differently, despite the shared event, and for some, it may lead to trauma.

Despite the wide range of events that can be potentially traumatic, if I was to compile a list of such events it would likely include any number of unexpected disaster events, accidents, physical violence, sexual assault, sexual abuse, childhood neglect, war, military combat experiences, natural disasters, mass casualty events, unexpected loss of a loved one, domestic and family violence, sustained bullying, poverty, invasive medical procedures, acts of terrorism, witnessing violence, emotional abuse or coercive control, and near-death experiences. Trauma in childhood can have disproportionate effects, meaning that events such as having a parent with enduring mental illness or substance use, parental incarceration, or acrimonious divorce are also known to be potentially traumatic. Across the lifespan, experiences such as structural racism or discrimination, financial stress, housing eviction, and climate change may all also lead to trauma.

Caruth describes trauma as an overwhelming experience that resists integration or expression (Caruth, 2016). This is important because we can experience potentially traumatic events, but if we have ways to integrate the experience into our narrative of the world or ways to express our emotional responses, the lasting impacts may be lessened. This helps to understand that not all potentially traumatic events are experienced in ways that lead to trauma.

There are different ways to categorise or describe trauma

There are many different types of trauma, some of which have been academically or clinically named or grouped and some of which haven't. Some of the groupings relate to the types of events and others to the types of effects. For example, there are known differences between trauma from environmental events (including accidents, disasters, and events) compared to interpersonal events between people. There are also known differences in effect between 'single incident trauma events' (one-off events) and 'cumulative trauma events' (repeated events).

Trauma that occurs from a single event or an environmental cause can have long-lasting effects on people, including a loss of trust in the predictability of life and the development of post-traumatic stress disorder (PTSD). However, the effects of traumas that occur with intent or in relationships, or over sustained periods of time, can be more complex. That is, they may be less linked specifically to reminders or thoughts of what happened and more woven into many aspects of people's lives. These can be called *complex trauma*. Complex trauma results from trauma exposure that occurs repeatedly, usually over a period of time, including childhood abuse, neglect, or interpersonal violence. The repeated nature of these experiences and their relational components means that people may experience sustained difficulties with self-regulation, relationships, and trust. People who have experienced complex trauma are also most likely to access healthcare services and receive care or treatment that does not address their needs or that is retraumatising. There is a lot to say about complex trauma, but maybe the most important thing is to recognise that how it develops and impacts is *complex*. It often also feels complex to the person who lives with it. The compounding effects of multiple events can make it hard to identify or articulate trauma when it is complex. For example, if you experience an assault as a young person, this is a single-event trauma. But if you are also living in a family where you experience neglect and a lack of love and care so that when you are assaulted there is no one to talk about it with or identify reparative actions, then this may actually be the more significant impacting trauma, but it is harder to explain or pinpoint. It may also impact you in ways that feel more complex. Your triggers may be more relational and linked to needs being met and a sense of care. There may be a devaluing of self. That means there is an acceptance or lack of recognition of neglect in future relationships which eventually leaves you more susceptible to further harm. It is not that in the moment of single-event harm you don't recognise it for what it is, but perhaps the relational cues leading up to that moment were impacted by trauma, as is the recovery. In this example, cumulative trauma creates complex effects, and the precipitating event becomes blurred.

Relational trauma occurs within relationships, usually families, and encompasses experiences of maltreatment, violence, abuse, neglect, serious and pervasive disruptions in caregiving, and abrupt separation or traumatic loss. Relational trauma can also refer to patterns of attachment interaction from caregiver to child that are intrusive, confusing, have a lack of warmth or soothing, or are antagonistic. These types of trauma are not discrete but are ways of describing and understanding experiences. Therefore, relational traumas can also be cumulative if there are repeated relational events or dynamics which compound each other; for example, people may experience multiple forms of violence or abuse in one relationship or various relationships. Relational traumas can also be *developmental* if they disrupt the stability and consistency required for development, and they can be *complex* if they lead to lifelong disturbances of how the self is understood. They can also be *intergenerational* or *transgenerational*. Nearly all types of trauma, however, have attributes related to disruption of how we see and understand ourselves in relation to the world and other people.

This book tries to consider all types of trauma, but if you notice a leaning towards more examples from interpersonal, complex, or relational forms of trauma than one-off disaster events, this is for a number of reasons. The first is that the (so-called) 'Big-T' one-off-a-very-obviously-bad-thing-happened traumas are more well understood, articulable, and apparent. They are largely not contentious or overlooked. The (so-called) 'little-t' traumas associated with cumulative or indirectly experienced events or exposure to abusive dynamics or childhood maltreatment are the ones that have been historically unrecognised or acknowledged in society. They are the ones that are often not documented in people's medical records and not able to be clearly explained or talked about. Yet they are also the ones that frequently impact upon healthcare interactions and require movements like Trauma Informed Care to ensure they are understood and recognised. Trauma that develops in relationships impacts relationships, including healthcare ones. I have used examples of these types of trauma a lot to try to demonstrate the less visible and more easily misunderstood ways that trauma can impact upon nursing and midwifery practice. However, I don't think any type of trauma is worse or more significant than others.

Part of understanding trauma and the roles it plays in our lives, our communities, and the world is recognising that there are complex ways that trauma memories live on in our bodies, our minds, and the present and are passed on through families and cultures. Some categories of trauma that have been defined are listed in Table 1.1.

Early life traumas or adversity experienced during childhood are sometimes referred to as *adverse childhood experiences* (ACE). In the 1990s, a landmark study on ACEs reported longitudinally on 17,000 people in the United States, linking their ACEs to their subsequent adult health (Felitti et al., 1998). The study found that exposure to ACEs had a powerful impact on adult mental and physical health. A strong relationship was identified between the number of ACEs and the presence of disease conditions associated with the leading causes of death in adults. ACEs were determined to be 'dose-dependent', meaning that the more you have, the more challenges are likely. Since the original study, there has been a lot of research which confirms and expands on the health and social implications of childhood adversity.

Table 1.1 Types of trauma

Single incident trauma	Trauma associated with a one-off shocking or distressing event, such as an act of violence or an environmental disaster
Interpersonal trauma	Trauma associated with actions of other people or within relationships, such as physical, emotional, or sexual violence, often impacting people's sense of safety and trust in others
Complex trauma	Repeated exposure to traumatic events or dynamics, often of an invasive, interpersonal nature, leading to long-term complex effects on emotional and psychological health
Relational trauma	Trauma associated with experiences and dynamics within key attachment or family relationships, including neglect, sustained misattunement, manipulation, betrayal, abandonment, or abuse
Attachment trauma	Trauma resulting from disruptions in the bond between an infant or child and their primary caregiver, affecting the developing sense of safety, security, and self
Betrayal trauma	Trauma associated with events where someone who should be trusted, such as a family member or person in a position of power, betrays assumptions of trust and safety
Intergenerational trauma	Trauma experienced across generations. The effects of trauma may be 'passed down' from one generation to the next without exposure to the initial events through behaviours, beliefs, and patterns within families
Cumulative trauma	The accumulation of multiple traumatic experiences over time, which can have a compounded effect on an individual's mental and emotional well-being
Adverse childhood experiences	Potentially traumatic events which occur during childhood. Inclusive of abuse, neglect, disrupted caregiving, or social disadvantage

ACEs are typically categorized as child abuse and neglect (including physical, sexual and emotional abuse, physical and emotional neglect), as well as household challenges such as exposure to family violence, living with a family member with mental illness or substance use disorder, parental divorce, incarceration of a household member, or living in poverty (Felitti et al., 1998). It is important to know that identifying ACEs was an approach developed for research purposes to identify the impacts of childhood trauma across the population, rather than to determine exactly how events impact individuals. Therefore, not everyone who experiences ACEs will have adverse health outcomes. ACEs are influenced by cultural, social, environmental, and economic factors that also affect health.

Box 1.2: Intergenerational transmission of trauma

Trauma can be passed across generations in various ways. There are traumatic events that occur across generations (either from sustained exposure or replicated patterns); for example, repeated trauma impacts multiple generations or occurs across generations, with multiple generations exposed to the same trauma. This is a continuation of trauma across generations. There are also families or communities where patterns play out; for example, if someone experienced violence as a child, then because of their framework for relationships, they may enter violent relationships as an adult, and then their children may also experience violence. This is a replication of trauma across generations. Then there are traumatic effects which are passed down without exposure to the traumatic events. It is not known exactly how the trauma of a parent or caregiver can be transmitted to a child or subsequent generation. It likely occurs in multiple ways. What is known is that people in subsequent generations from a primary trauma may display effects of trauma despite not having experienced the events directly. This is observed in families who have experienced war or traumatic loss, but it can also occur in any relational trauma.

My work with parents and infants has made me most interested in the relational processes by which a blurring of self and other leads to trauma of the caregiver becoming incorporated into the self of the infant. Infants develop in close reliance upon adults, usually parents. They learn from what adults tell them is true, but they also learn from what they see over and over, and they learn who they are intersubjectively. Intersubjectivity refers to a crucial task undertaken by caregivers when they reflect infants' internal states back to them through empathic mirroring, to inform the cohesion of a sense of 'self' (Kohut, 1971; Schore, 2009). For example, 'I see your repeated delight in me, and over time I learn that I can be delightful'. This mirroring is also bidirectional. The infant mirrors the caregivers' internal states and relies on the caregiver to organise theirs. When there is trauma present, infants match the rhythmic structures of the caregiver's dysregulated arousal states across many moments and internalise them as their own. The developing infant brain can seemingly imprint not only the overwhelming affective states of the caregiver's trauma but also the unconscious coping mechanisms (such as dissociation) that the caregiver has developed to manage. Over time, the infant essentially takes on the effects of trauma, without linking these effects to a precipitant.

We can also absorb trauma like we do culture or any other unspoken teachings we gain from family or community about what life is, who we are, and what we can expect. Like many aspects of our culture, there are many things never directly explained that we just know. We may not remember how we learnt how to act, how to move, what to do, what is acceptable and not acceptable, and what is scary and safe in this world, but we learnt it through what we were told and even more so what we saw. And sometimes what we saw contradicted what we were told.

A common and universal parenting instinct is to keep children safe. When trauma has occurred for the parent, that drive can be amplified because assumptions of safety have been shattered. This can play out in various ways for parents who have experienced trauma, including wanting their kids to be independent or self-sufficient from an early age. But it can also sometimes mean they work very hard to keep their children safer than they ever were. They may never leave their child with anyone, they make sure to pick them up from places always, they never let them walk alone, they may ask lots of questions about safety and reinforce the need to be careful, and they may warn them of things. The paradox is that these extra efforts for safety are also reinforcing a constant message of danger. As the child develops, presumably safely, they are learning fear and lack of safety at the forefront of their experience. Alongside messaging about fear and danger, this can also reduce joy, imagination, and freedom if safety is always the priority. In this way, despite being well-cared for and protected, they can absorb the effects of the trauma of the parent. If we then imagine how they, the children, might make sense of their fear and uneasy feelings as adults, they would search their minds to figure out where this response comes from and find nothing, because they have always been safe and the traumatic events that led to these feelings were not theirs. This is a minor example, and of course it is good to keep children safe and parents who work hard to give their children a better childhood than they had are to be commended. But it's an example of how words and actions can paradoxically teach the very things we are trying to protect children from. And once the feeling is passed on, it becomes the person's, and it becomes very hard to become aware of what emotions we have absorbed from others.

Finally, it is also important to identify the role that epigenetics may play in intergenerational trauma. Epigenetics is the study of how genes can be expressed differently based on the environment. So, exposure to trauma may lead to gene expressions which can influence what genes are expressed, repressed, or enhanced in the next generation, without altering DNA. Some of the classic examples of attempts to demonstrate this in research contexts are through using smells and pain to teach fear conditioning, demonstrating that mice two generations later still react to certain smells with fear, despite having never felt the pain themselves. In humans, studies of populations who have survived famine similarly demonstrate altered appetite and fat storage generations later. Epigenetics is adaptive; it facilitates survival through the learnings of ancestors. It is possible that the effects of the fear and betrayal of trauma can also be passed on in this way.

How events are experienced is important for trauma

How events are experienced is crucial to whether they become traumatic. Potentially Traumatic Events are commonly experienced as inescapable or overwhelming of people's capacity to cope, often also involving fear or betrayal. Events can be inescapable because of a person's age or vulnerability, or because of their environment or circumstances. They can also be inescapable because of dynamics of power and control. How events are experienced can be impacted by many things, including age, frame of understanding, culture, spiritual beliefs, social and interpersonal support, opportunities for meaning making and reflection, previous exposure to trauma, coping strategies, and so on.

Usually trauma renders people helpless, either in the moment or over time. For some people, trauma may develop not from one moment of extreme fear but because of cumulative or sustained dynamics which lead to a loss of self or agency over time. Trauma usually develops from events or circumstances which fracture assumptions of safety. The experience can be extraordinary and shatter assumptions of safety in one moment of terror or horror, but it can also be very ordinary; for example, many people may find themselves stuck in domestic situations which lead to a slow degradation of power and agency, leading to self-blame and shame. Sometimes events shatter what assumptions people held about the world (for example, 'the world is mostly safe and people are mostly good and kind'), and at other times, particularly within families or relationships, the shattering is woven into how they understand the world (for example, 'you can't trust anyone and everything is dangerous'); both are difficult in different ways but either way there is often a disconnection from self, from others, fear, and either intrusive memories or fracturing of consciousness to avoid intrusive memories.

Box 1.3: Trauma in adulthood

James worked for the Military for 7 years. Here he reflects on his experience

> It was what I always wanted to do. I joined straight from school, and I thought I'd be there for my whole career, my whole life. After completing my training, I got sent overseas with a special unit. It's hard to explain what I saw over there. Only the other guys who were there really get it. There was an incredible camaraderie, we had been through this life changing experience together, seen things humans should never see, participated in things that would horrify you. I drank a lot at first when I got back to try not to remember, but mostly now I just see it in my dreams.
>
> I got injured and I was medically discharged from the army in 2017. That's when things got hard. You are probably thinking that I have trauma from all the things I saw … maybe I do. But the worst bit for me has been the sense that I don't matter. That I am no longer useful. It feels like I got kicked out of my family. The only place I had ever belonged. I was part of something, I belonged, I was with people who got it, who got me. But what family kicks you out when you are injured? It makes me wonder what the point of it was. Why did I fight? It makes me wonder if I made the right choices in doing the things I did. So yeah, I do have trauma, I'm a traumatised war veteran, that's probably the easiest way to describe it, but it's not just from the war.

In this example, various PTEs are identified. James saw and participated in things that continue to intrude on his subconscious, but there is a relational trauma apparent also. Relational trauma is expressed in how he felt to be discharged from the army and the lost sense of belonging, purpose, and identity which led to a questioning of self and trust.

New 'types' of trauma emerge all the time

Events that are potentially traumatic are socially defined and are also able to change over time. To use a recent example, during the global Covid-19 pandemic, talk of collective and shared trauma was widespread, alongside individual and familial experiences of loss and fear. Nurses working through the pandemic experienced trauma from caring for dying people, isolation, and worries for their own families, as did whole communities who felt betrayed by their governments and feared for their lives.

Climate change is another example. The global climate crisis is not a potentially traumatic event that may result in trauma for some people under certain circumstances, but rather a new form of trauma that pervades the circumstances of modern life. The mass threat of the changing climate and the sense that it has already overwhelmed our capacity to cope or adapt is characteristic of trauma. Climate trauma, like Covid-19 trauma, is both personal and cultural. Unlike Covid-19, climate trauma goes beyond immediate events which can be contained in the past; it fundamentally alters the world and our perceptions of it. As a result, young people across the world are experiencing trauma linked to hopelessness about the future and a sense of betrayal from adults and governments who should have been protective (Hickman et al., 2021).

Iatrogenic trauma and retraumatisation in healthcare

Sometimes trauma is caused in healthcare. Trauma that occurs in care is known as iatrogenic trauma. People can experience harm directly through medical procedures or scary experiences. Other times, they may experience more subtle forms of trauma through fear, betrayal, helplessness, or coercion. While the events that cause distress in healthcare may not always be avoidable, as with any trauma, the impacts relate to how events are experienced. Experiences of illness, injury or pain, and medication or treatment can be traumatic due to potential loss of control, loss of hope, or loss of touch with reality. Trauma can also occur from procedures that are painful, emergency situations, sustained treatments that make people sick, or watching family members suffer. Often experiences are amplified by fear or a sense of betrayal. People may feel betrayed that they should have been cared for and they weren't or that they needed help and it wasn't received. We might consider something that happened in care as 'minor' but it seems to have had a big effect on someone. Or we might be very clear that what happened 'had to happen' to save their life or keep them safe. But as with all trauma, it doesn't matter what the reason was that it occurred; it matters how it was experienced by the person. This means that what is iatrogenically traumatic to someone may not be anticipatable. I saw a woman who became ill after an anaesthetic and was on bedrest post operatively to avoid falls. While she was cared for and safe, she thought she might die and felt nobody helped her. She felt her hospital bed had become her coffin and months later she has flashbacks of the blank faces of nurses looking down on her. She is left with is a memory of being alone and scared.

The dynamics of healthcare can also replicate power dynamics of trauma experiences and be retraumatising for people who have already experienced trauma in their lives. Retraumatisation refers to circumstances which lead a person to re-experience a previously traumatic event. They may be conscious this is occurring, or they may unconsciously re-experience the same emotions and thoughts of that event without clearly delineating the past from present. Retraumatisation means that the experience of care can reenact the same dynamics of trauma, replicating harm. This can occur from overt things, such as being held down or having intrusive investigations without adequate pain relief or sedation. But it can also occur through aspects of care that seem benign. For example, the power dynamics inherent in many care interactions, the powerlessness of hospitalisation or particularly smells or sensations.

Exposure to potentially traumatic events is common

Exposure to potentially traumatic events is common. Statistics are commonly spouted of 60% to 70% of all adults having been exposed to traumatic events. This is both helpful and unhelpful. It is helpful to recognise that exposure to traumatic events is not a rare occurrence or something that only impacts a very small amount of people who may be accessing or receiving care. It is helpful for raising awareness of trauma and for rallying funding, organisational commitments, and public health approaches. It is unhelpful in that it can take away from recognising the severity and impacts of trauma upon many people.

Some groups and individuals may be more 'vulnerable' to trauma. While trauma affects all demographics of people, it also disproportionately impacts people based on access to resources, safety, supports, and socio-economic positioning. Understanding vulnerability to sustained impacts of trauma is important for nurses and midwives as the impact of traumatic life experiences is not always visible at the time of the event but may affect people's lives later. This relates directly to experiences in care (such as intrusive interventions or treatments) and experiences that lead people to access care (such as assaults, injuries, or accidents).

It is likely that nurses and midwives working in all areas of healthcare will be providing care to people who have experienced trauma. In some areas of healthcare, prevalence rates are higher still, such as in populations of disadvantaged young people, people with mental illness or substance use, or homelessness. In public mental health services, for example, prevalence estimates are 90% of people who access services have experienced physical, sexual, or psychological trauma in their lifetime.

Health and social service providers have also known to have a higher prevalence of lifetime trauma than the general population. This is important when identifying how best to support the workforce, as people who have experienced one or more traumatic events in their own lives are also at higher risk of developing secondary traumatic stress resulting from helping people with trauma or distress. Many people are drawn to helping professions such as nursing and midwifery because of trauma experiences in their own lives. It is therefore likely that nurses and midwives working in all areas of healthcare will be providing care to people who have experienced trauma and may also have their own experiences of trauma. Having a solid understanding of trauma is therefore important for beginning to think about what it means to be trauma informed.

To conclude this chapter, it is important to acknowledge the challenges in defining and describing trauma. Exposure to potentially traumatic events that usually involve direct or indirect fear, betrayal, loss, horror or control is common. However, people will experience these events in differing ways based on a variety of internal, external, and social factors. At times people may be left with lasting psychological effects which impact their functioning or become woven into their way of seeing the world and themselves. This is trauma. Trauma can be relational, environmental, intergenerational, iatrogenic, or difficult to categorise or describe. These are all trauma.

References

Caruth, C. (2016). *Unclaimed experience: Trauma, narrative, and history* (Twentieth Anniversary edition). Johns Hopkins University Press.

Felitti, V. J., Anda, R. F., Nordenberg, D., Williamson, D. F., Spitz, A. M., Edwards, V., Koss, M. P., & Marks, J. S. (1998). Relationship of childhood abuse and household dysfunction to many of the leading causes of death in adults. *American Journal of Preventive Medicine, 14*(4), 245–258. https://doi.org/10.1016/S0749-3797(98)00017-8

Hickman, C., Marks, E., Pihkala, P., Clayton, S., Lewandowski, R. E., Mayall, E. E., Wray, B., Mellor, C., & Van Susteren, L. (2021). Climate anxiety in children and young people and their beliefs about government responses to climate change: A global survey. *The Lancet Planetary Health, 5*(12), e863–e873. https://doi.org/10.1016/S2542-5196(21)00278-3

Kohut, H. (1971). *The analysis of the self: A systematic approach to the psychoanalytic treatment of narcissistic personality disorders.* International Universities Press.

Schore, A. N. (2009). Relational trauma and the developing right brain: An interface of psychoanalytic self psychology and neuroscience. *Annals of the New York Academy of Sciences, 1159*(1), 189–203. https://doi.org/10.1111/j.1749-6632.2009.04474.x

Substance Abuse and Mental Health Services Administration [SAMHSA]. (2014). *SAMHSA's concept of trauma and guidance for a trauma-informed approach* (HHS Publication No. SMA14-4884). U.S. Department of Health and Human Services. https://www.samhsa.gov/mental-health/trauma-violence/trauma-informed-approaches-programs

2 How trauma affects people

People respond to potentially traumatic events or circumstances in a wide variety of ways. The most common response to trauma is resilience. People cope with, survive, and endure trauma all the time. However, alongside resilience, trauma can affect health, well-being, life, and functioning in overt ways, as well as ways that are not always visible to others or that the person themselves may not be aware of. Trauma can impact how people understand themselves and others, their experiences of the world, and core assumptions. It can also affect autonomic stress response systems, physical and mental health, and interactions with people and services. Traumatic effects differ across the lifespan, are impacted by other factors, supports, and resources in people's lives, and are related to the type of traumatic events or experiences that people experience.

Impacts differ based on exposure

There is increasing recognition that the timing of potentially traumatic events in people's lives can alter the lasting effects. This is perhaps similar to how it matters exactly what stage of pregnancy a pregnant person is exposed to a toxin because it will impact the development that is occurring at that time; the timing of trauma exposure differs based on our stage of emotional, cognitive, and social development. These are things that continue to develop the whole time we are alive. There is more and more research emerging about how trauma impacts during infancy, childhood, adolescence, adulthood, and older age. How trauma differs across the lifespan can be quite subtle, but also important.

Box 2.1: Examples of trauma impacts at different stages of life

Consider the following examples of how trauma impacts differently based on age of exposure:

   Matty experienced sexual abuse by a family friend when he was very young and before he could speak or really remember things. He knew about it because his family had found out at the time, but he was an infant and had no memory of the incidents. Throughout his life, he experienced pervasive body shame and low self-esteem, but it was hard for him to say if it was related to the trauma. He was plagued by a feeling that he was disgusting, although he couldn't identify where

---

DOI: 10.4324/9781003530770-4

this feeling had developed from. In his late 40s, he was required to have a colonoscopy. In the days before and after the procedure, he was disturbed by intense nightmares about his abuse as an infant. In the nightmares, he was watching the abuse take place and screaming at the perpetrator. Following the procedure, the nightmares persisted, and Matty started to experience more intense daily trauma symptoms. He wasn't sure if it was real or imagined.

Ray grew up in a household where there was violence from a young age. His parents went through a long and difficult divorce during his early childhood years and were violent towards each other, as well as Ray and his siblings. As an adult, Ray identifies that he never learnt how to get his needs met. He learnt very early on to suppress his own needs and be invisible to avoid conflict. He is fearful and hypervigilant about causing anyone any trouble. This has caused him great difficulty in his relationships as an adult.

Miranda experienced abuse by her stepfather from the age of 12 when he came into her life, until age 15 when she left home. In her late teens and early 20s, she took a lot of drugs and lived a risky lifestyle. In her late 20s, she got into exercise and began running marathons to cope. She met her husband and had two daughters. She got divorced when her daughters were 8 and 10. A couple of years later, she began dating a new partner. The age of her daughters and the presence of her new partner in the home brought up intense flashbacks of her abuse. She began drinking heavily and over the course of a couple of months lost her licence for drink-driving, could no longer practice as a health professional due to her charges, and broke up with her partner.

Sasha had a happy childhood. As a teenager, she developed severe cystic acne which led her to feel very self-conscious about her appearance. She became fixated on her skin and how horrible she must appear to others. She experienced extreme bullying at school and began to withdraw socially. Once her skin improved and she left school, things improved; however, as an adult, she still avoids mirrors or any situation where anyone may touch or see her skin.

Clara started a new relationship in her late 50s with a partner who became violent. She had previously been happily married, successful at work, and a parent to teenage children. The violent relationship lasted 5 years, during which time she felt she lost all sense of who she was. Prior to the relationship, she had felt reasonably comfortable in herself, had a good social network, and trusted people easily. After the relationship, she felt destabilised in every way. The things she thought she knew about herself and the world were no longer certain.

Pat was involved in a car accident in her early 70s where the driver of the other car died. Pat was not at fault, but she had a recurring sense that maybe it was her fault in some way. Following the accident, Pat withdrew from her community and became isolated. She experienced regular intrusive imagery of the accident and started taking daily pain medication to deal with her physical ailments and to numb her emotional pain. Her family thought that she had 'aged a lot' since the accident, but she did not tell them about her ongoing negative thoughts and moods as she did not want to burden them. She experienced increasing physical health complaints and started to wish she wasn't alive.

In the examples in Box 2.1, it is apparent that the stage of life and development that the person was at, at the time of trauma exposure, impacted the ways that it affected their sense of self and life. Early traumas were more woven into Matty and Ray's ways of thinking about themselves in ways that were difficult to articulate or recognise. Miranda's and Sasha's capacities to trust other people or perceive themselves through the eyes of others were altered, whereas for Clara and Pat, everything they thought they knew about themselves and the world was shattered. How trauma impacts people across the lifespan is not linear and is influenced by numerous factors; however, it is an important component of understanding trauma.

The effects of trauma are pervasive

While there are some 'common' ways trauma impacts people, it can also have very different and subtle impacts, regardless of when it occurs. People may think of themselves or the world differently, may have altered stress response systems, or may experience intrusive flashbacks or nightmares. Some common psychological effects include overwhelming stress, pervasive shame, negative self-image, changes in mood, fear and worry, mistrust, and distress. People may experience alterations to stress response systems leading to hyper-vigilance or dysregulation, dissociation, a disrupted sense of self, loss of cohesion of time and narrative, as well as interruptions to the language parts of the brain so that there are things that literally can't be spoken about. People, including children, may use forms of self-harm to distract themselves, soothe, feel alive, express distress, symbolise pain, resist control, or seek help. Social impacts can include disruptions to everyday life and relationships, an increase in coping strategies such as alcohol or drug use or self-harm, withdrawal, disconnection, and increased engagement in health, housing, criminal justice, and social services. Physical impacts can include exhaustion, insomnia or sleep disturbance, digestive issues, lowered immune function or chronic pain, and health conditions. The consequences of exposure to any form of trauma can be profound and lifelong. All trauma exposure is correlated to higher rates of mental health diagnosis and difficulty recovering or modulating distress, isolating from conflict, impaired ability to form or benefit from a social network, and interpretation of supportive efforts of others as threatening. This can mean that people respond unexpectedly to care and attempts to support them.

There are contradictions inherent to trauma. We may try to banish the thought of atrocities from our consciousness (Herman, 1992), while they may also refuse to be forgotten. Sometimes it is our attempts to banish trauma from consciousness that keeps it present in our lives. To live with trauma often involves complicated coping mechanisms that seek to minimise the power of trauma but can either directly impact our lives or inadvertently sustain trauma dynamics of shame and silencing. There are also frequently contradictions between not wanting to be defined by trauma and not being understood without knowing of it, wanting to be close to people to aid healing, and finding being in connection with others very difficult. There can be contradictions between states of arousal, feeling both numb and feeling too much, feeling shame about shame, forgetting some important things and being unable to forget others and so on.

Trauma can impact how people view themselves

Trauma commonly evokes feelings of betrayal, shame, guilt, and self-blame. People commonly hold conscious or unconscious persistent beliefs about themselves as diminished, defeated, or worthless. Trauma can shatter assumptions of safety and trust and alter the sense of self in relation to others. We all see ourselves, at least in part, by how we imagine others view us. The part of us considered the 'self' is socially constructed. It develops initially through repeated interactions with our primary caregivers through our first years of life and becomes formed based on how we imagine we look or seem to others, the way we imagine others judge us, and the feeling that results from this, for example, pride, disgust, delight, or shame.

While the moments that led to trauma are usually in the past, trauma can infiltrate the present. This occurs through warping of memory and time but also through these ways that trauma impacts the self. For example, people may internalise a version of the person who caused them trauma, sustaining trauma in the present through beliefs that they are unworthy, unsafe, unlovable, or disgusting. Exposure to trauma during childhood can alter the way that self-talk occurs. This doesn't mean hearing voices of perpetrators (although this can also be a remnant of trauma), but instead it refers to the way that we talk to ourselves, whether we are hyper-critical or shaming or blaming, for example. Essentially, you may survive abuse or relational trauma in the moment, but many people internalise an essence of the perpetrator entwined in their self. This may lead to internal harsh criticism of self or self-blame (*I always mess everything up. I am hopeless*) and, amongst other pathways of trauma, keeps the past alive in the present.

The self is not one part of the brain but is built of numerous pathways across sections, so it takes time to form and solidify and can be difficult to alter. Schore (Schore, 2002, 2009) has done a lot of work and writing about relational trauma and the developing brain and self. He describes that the early social environment of infants, which is most commonly mediated by the primary caregiver(s), influences how the neural pathways of the brain are established in relation to regulation and the development of a known and felt 'self'. The parts of the brain that Schore identifies process social and emotional information beneath awareness. Trauma can therefore become woven into our selves in ways that are hard to isolate.

Memories and self are linked, meaning we build a sense of ourselves based on our capacity to recall times and circumstances. However, trauma disrupts the cohesion or perception of memory and can contribute to disturbances in self-organisation. We may lose a sense of who we are or who we have been. Trauma can also more literally alter how we perceive our bodies, altering proprioception and sense of self in space. When people have experienced pain and powerlessness within their body, it makes sense to be able to separate from conscious awareness of sensations and connection. This can be a learnt mechanism of surviving sustained or overwhelming sensations but can lead to a sense of 'dis-embodiment' or detachment from self.

Trauma creates a paradox of shame

Often what makes experiences of trauma have sustained effects is related to elements of shame or self-blame. In adulthood or single-incident events, this may be linked to thoughts of what should have happened or what we should have done or not done. Trauma that occurs in childhood can be internalised by children because of their developmental stage and the dynamics of childhood trauma. They may believe it occurred because of something they have done or haven't done. Similarly, in adulthood, we often replay situations in our minds repeatedly, trying to make sense of what we did or did not do. We may feel shame about how we are impacted by events or because of traumatic events themselves. Shame about oneself can be a significant and debilitating component of trauma. As Dorahy describes, 'Chronically traumatised individuals feel shame not only for what has happened to them, but for who they are' (Dorahy et al., 2013). This shame runs deep and defies reassurance.

Shame is one of the key mechanisms through which trauma effects sustain themselves. We feel shame for whatever happened, and we feel shame for our responses to it. We might feel shame that we let it happen or that we didn't stop it from happening, or we might feel shame for our ongoing inability to 'get over it' or for ways that we respond in the present that are linked to trauma. We might feel shame for the things we do to cope with trauma or to reduce our distress from trauma. We may feel shame for things that happened in the moment of trauma – did we freeze and not fight back? Did we run away and not help others? Did we make decisions that left us vulnerable to the event, or did we trust the wrong people? Did we make too much noise or not enough noise? Were we told it was our fault? Often, in complex trauma, the trauma is so woven into the construction of our 'self' that instead of shame linked to a moment or a response, we feel shame for who we are. This is a deep and powerful form of shame which can be expressed in many ways. We may feel like we are weird or critically flawed in some way. We may feel like if people knew the real us, they would be horrified. We may feel we have to perform to try to fit in, or we may feel perpetually different or strange. It is a great burden to go through life having to work to hide yourself or parts of yourself, 'masking' or distracting or being incredible in other ways to ensure people don't see the bits of you that are broken. And the paradox is, our attempts to hide the things that we feel shame for, so we don't activate shame, keep us disconnected and hidden and hiding. Perhaps we avoid getting close to people in case they see that we are flawed in connection, and then as a result we have no close connections and feel lonely and disconnected, perpetuating the shame feeling. Or perhaps we hide our body because of things that have happened to it or ways it is, which means we don't seek help for things we need for our body, and then difficulties escalate. Shame is such a powerful controller of our ways of being, thinking, and feeling. Shame likes to hide in the shadows where the light can't reach it. It goes to great lengths to avoid light touching it, because when we bring shame out into the light, it loses its power. This is the paradox of shame and trauma. Trauma creates shame, and then shame keeps trauma hidden; shame creates problems for us but also stops us from seeking help or talking about those problems, which creates more shame. It's like a dodgy pyramid scheme.

When people experience shame for parts of their selves, they may develop defence mechanisms to hide these parts. These can include over-accommodation, aggression, constructed identities (or a 'false self'), or changeable identities. Some of these mechanisms sound extreme, but they can also be highly adaptive and not noticeable. For example, people may become 'chameleons' – adapting to any context or relationship, altering their self slightly to blend in or go unnoticed. This can, of course, be something we all do sometimes, but for some people who have experienced trauma, it can be consistent and unconscious.

Shame is thought to have developed to serve an important evolutionary purpose for humans by helping us maintain social cohesion. Shame acts as a social regulator, discouraging behaviours that could harm relationships or the stability of a group. As relational creatures, being part of a group is crucial for survival. Shame also serves a purpose similar to pain; it is an alarm bell of potential social harm by anticipating possible negative reactions of others towards us. Like pain, which warns us of physical harm, shame warns us of potential social harm. While what is considered shameful differs across groups and contexts, shame itself is thought to be a universal emotion. Shame can be both personal and social and is associated with how we see ourselves to be seen by others. Shame can be reinforced by external social forces such as cultural or religious expectations, rigid institutions, or strict interpersonal dynamics. Shame is associated with emotions and experiences, such as powerlessness, disgust, self-contempt, and despair, and is further complicated by its self-perpetuating nature, where confusingly we can feel shame about experiencing shame. Shame can also be anticipatory; this means that persistent concerns about the possibility of shame can also be destructive. Many people live with a sustained sense of anticipation of shame. They may engage in avoidance or other strategies to avoid the activation of shame which can lead to a cycle. De Young describes this debilitating cycle of shame: 'What they live with is not shame, but "what it costs them to keep from falling into shame' (DeYoung, 2015, p. 19). Shame hides trauma. Shame is associated with trauma.

I recall a woman I was seeing for perinatal anxiety who looked outwardly composed, well dressed, hair done nicely, socially and professionally successful, yet described a history of childhood sexual abuse. She also described feeling 'dead inside … if you looked inside me, you'd be surprised to find a black hole of nothingness'. I recall her saying this with a smile on her face, her appearance a distraction from what she saw as the great abyss of nothingness inside her.

People often feel shame about parts of themselves or their lives that are unexpectedly revealed, but they can also feel shame about things that they desperately don't want to be revealed. Shame can be linked to our bodies or our minds, but shame can also be linked to our whole self. Wille (Wille, 2014) calls this 'the shame of existing'. The shame of existing is so woven with the self that it is not about who you are or what you have done or are doing but is linked just to the fact that you are. Rather than trying to hide or conceal this shame, people may instead just want to disappear. Encountering people with this intensity of shame can evoke difficult feelings for us as nurses and midwives. Shame invites us to absorb it. For example, if someone feels unworthy of being cared for, we can start to feel shame about trying to care.

Silence also contributes to shame. This can become a cycle. Things are shameful to talk about, so they aren't spoken of, and then shame grows. Trauma is often hard to talk about because it is inherently shocking and uncomfortable. It requires us to think beyond the boundaries of what we like to believe about the world and people. There has always been a tendency to push traumatic events not only out of individual consciousness but also out of collective social consciousness, as to acknowledge trauma requires acceptance of human capabilities for evil and vulnerability (Herman, 1992). This creates a 'dialectic' of trauma, in that people who experience trauma and society, both simultaneously, can't bear to acknowledge the reality of the events while also needing them to be acknowledged and spoken of for healing or reparative action. As a society and within relationships, denial of trauma is not uncommon. When perpetrators of trauma, violence, or abuse hold power and are influential, silencing, shaming, and discrediting trauma survivors becomes acceptable.

I heard John Briere once say that 'avoidance is the best way to sustain pain'. He was talking about the ways we get stuck in trauma, but he was also saying how as a society avoidance is the most acceptable strategy for psychological pain. We can listen to people express distress or pain for a short period, and then we want them to stop. And subsequently, pain does not get processed, and we collude as individuals and society to avoid it. Thereby sustaining it.

Shame is a common part of trauma experiences for many individuals. Shame may underpin 'symptoms' of trauma. Shame is a feeling and thought process which focuses not on what happened (e.g. 'an awful thing happened to me') or an individual's actions (e.g. 'I did something awful') but rather condemns the self (e.g. 'I am an awful person'). Shame stops the integration of traumatic memories into a person's framework of understanding themselves, preventing recovery. Shame is particularly linked to experiences of powerlessness, humiliation, and loss of control within relational traumas.

Trauma can impact upon relationships

Trauma can impact people's capacity to trust other people. This is especially true when trauma occurs within relationships. It is an assumption to see this lack of trust as a cognitive error, because it makes sense not to trust people if people who you should have been able to trust hurt you. However, a lack of trust in other people can affect daily functioning. Society is built upon a required degree of trust. A lack of trust may impact through being overly self-reliant to the extent that people can't or won't ever seek any help or support due to beliefs that other people will betray or harm them. It may also impact through communication challenges associated with being unable to clearly express feelings or needs. This may have been learnt over time because it was unsafe or ineffective to express needs or emotions. People may feel their needs are a burden to others or will have negative consequences, or they may have learnt to shut off awareness of even having any emotions or needs. They may have not been given language as children to express or recognise their needs. Having no needs or emotions may be a survival strategy, but it can be quite challenging to be in any form of relationship with someone who has learnt to function in this way. It can make other people feel wary or uncomfortable, it can cause tension, or it can leave people vulnerable to exploitation and further harm. Alternatively, people who have experienced trauma may have heightened emotional responses which can cause conflict. A lack of trust can also be expressed through aggressive or anti-social behaviour.

Trauma can impact relationships in surface-level ways where people are experienced as 'needy' or 'prickly' or 'too much' or 'too distant', or it can make people avoid getting close to other people to minimise pain and to hide their trauma. On a deeper level, it can disrupt the nature of attachment bonds, where people may perpetually feel insecure even in trusting and loving relationships, leading to excessive worry, need for reassurance, or emotional detachment.

It is important to also see that trauma can make people deeply value safe and reliable relationships. If trauma doesn't get in the way of developing and sustaining such connections, they may be treasured and deeply healing. But it takes time to build trust, and there may be a residual hypervigilance to ruptures.

Trauma can be ongoing

Much of the talk about trauma focuses on events that have passed and left a lasting impact. But trauma can also exist or be perpetuated in the present. To use a common example, nurses and midwives may be working with patients currently experiencing domestic and family violence (DFV). It is essential to recognise the dynamics of power and control that perpetuate experiences like DFV, beyond an incident focused view of any overt acts of violence. DFV involves the perpetrator exercising power and control through emotional, physical, or sexual violence, as well as the experience of coercion, stalking, and psychological aggression. Awareness of trauma means consideration of the dynamics that impede disclosure of DFV and that keep people in such relationships. DFV can occur for anyone but can also occur on a background of other forms of complex trauma that have altered people's expectations of other people, capacity to consciously recognise dynamics of abuse, or learnt drives to attach to people who are simultaneously unsafe. However, viewing people who experience DFV as vulnerable is also problematic as it minimises recognition of the powerful dynamics of coercion and power that maintain violence. Responsibility for DFV should rest with the perpetrator and not the person experiencing it. This can be confronting and uncomfortable to accept, with societal attitudes to DFV often contributing to its impacts upon people. DFV is just one way that people may be presenting to healthcare while continuing to experience violence. It provides an important opportunity for nurses and midwives to hold awareness of how trauma gets enacted and sustained within relationships.

Box 2.2: The dynamics of DFV

In this example, Brenda reflects on her experiences of the dynamics of DFV.

> I met my ex-partner at work. I didn't pay much attention to him at first because he wasn't really my type. He was kind of nerdy and I much preferred to date men who were a bit more edgy. That seems silly to say now. He seemed interested in me. Eventually I just decided to say yes when he asked me out. At first, he was … fine. There were times when he made me a bit uncomfortable or seemed a bit critical, but I just ignored or dismissed those. I convinced myself he was good for me and that I was making a mature choice. We stayed together for 4 years. At first, he was just a bit controlling; he would tell me who I could go out with and what I should wear and make comments about my appearance. When I say it like that it seems obvious, but somehow it just… wasn't. It was little comments buried in amongst normality. Not even normality, better than my normality, he would buy nice things, take me on nice trips, make me feel like I owed him. He wasn't aggressive or violent; we had a nice time together in lots of ways. It wasn't all bad, which is another thing I didn't really understand until I'd lived it – it doesn't have to be all bad to be abusive. I always thought I would never be the type of person to be in an abusive relationship but what I realised is that it can take a long time to even realise that is what it is. He had a way of undermining my confidence so that over time I couldn't tell what was normal anymore. He told me I was fat, that I smelled, that I was weird, that I was boring, that I was lucky to have him. He wanted me to quit my job, not see my friends, not see my family. He wanted me to not talk about things that made him uncomfortable, like feminism or anything political. Somehow he managed to convince me that he was right about all the things that he said about me and so I never told anyone around me any of it. He seemed harmless to everyone else, a bit weird maybe but he'd found the perfect place to hide his abuse – beneath a very usual seeming exterior. But within the 'normality' of everyday life, he had woven a way of controlling me and everything I did. And by the time

I realised that, I couldn't believe it was true. I felt so embarrassed actually. It's embarrassing to be hurt by someone you love. It is hard to understand that you can love someone who hurts you.

When you ask me about what parts of it traumatised me, it's hard to explain. I have no physical wounds. And my life now is good. I got out before I was tied to him forever. But it has still left scars. Deep scars on bits of me that are hard to talk about. On some level I still believe what he told me. Or at least I turn those thoughts over in my mind and wonder if they are true – am I fat? Am I smelly? Am I boring? I can tell myself logically that he was abusive and he said all those things to manipulate and control me but on a bad day I still find myself wearing extra perfume or trying to think of great conversation starters. I can continue to punish myself by wondering if maybe it wasn't abuse and he was just telling me the truth. That's what he used to say to me, "You can at least trust me to tell you the truth". I still have nightmares about him often and I wake up sweating. If I leave the kitchen messy, I hear his voice telling me how disgusting I am. If I wear sneakers, I hear him tell me how stupid I look in those shoes. And this is over 5 years later. Plus, maybe the other legacy is that he was a health professional. His job was to help people. I find that very hard to get past. I don't like to see male doctors anymore. I know that isn't fair as they aren't all him, but I lost trust in my own ability to know who is trustworthy and who isn't, or perhaps I lost trust in the idea that some people are trustworthy and some people aren't. I used to think I was a really good judge of character. But now I need to take other precautions, mainly I just don't put myself in vulnerable positions with any man if I can avoid it. Just in case.

In Brenda's story, dynamics of control and power are evident, as well as the pervasive way they altered how she viewed herself and the world. Although the relationship is now in the past, she describes ways that the abuse continues to impact her feelings of safety and trust in the world and her own capacity to know. She has internalised a voice that continues to keep the abuse alive in her present.

It is impossible to clearly summarise exactly how trauma impacts people. Patterns of experiences across communities and groups show that alterations occur in how people see themselves, the world, and other people. These alterations make sense in the context of adaptation to a world that is experienced as unsafe, untrustworthy, or risky. However, the ways we adjust perception or understanding to account for trauma or to minimise the likelihood of further or ongoing harm can themselves cause difficulties and become part of the ways that trauma exists in the present.

Resilience is a part of trauma

In addition to recognising the potential for trauma to impact upon health and be implicated in illness, trauma awareness also requires recognition of the relationship between trauma and resilience and people's capacity to recover.

I am reminded of when I went to Rio De Janeiro in Brazil at a time when the city was experiencing a lot of violence. There were many warnings about the lack of safety and the need to remain vigilant at all times to a possible threat. While there, I spoke to a taxi driver who had lived in Rio all his life. I asked him how he copes with the constant feeling of being unsafe. He told me that it is like any other problem in life; somehow you have to continue to live your life and find joy, despite the bad things. He described how he refuses to let the violence take away his freedom to go out, to have fun, and to be happy. People often do find ways to find safety within ongoing trauma and sustain connection in environments that are unsafe.

Resilience is not distinct from trauma, as often people who experience trauma also display incredible resilience. There are many definitions of resilience; they all involve something along the lines of 'bouncing back' or adapting to adversity or trauma or stress. However, resilience is not so much about recovering to the place you were prior to the adversity, but also about coping and growing within the context of adversity. Resilience is a capacity present in everyone. We all have the capacity to adapt to stress and adversity, to enable coping. It is not the same as being tough or not feeling sadness, fear, anger, or distress. Resilience encompasses both positive and negative trajectories that occur after adversity and is a dynamic and interactional concept. That is, resilience is influenced by environmental factors, community and social networks, and social determinants of health and has the capacity to change over time.

People can be resilient in some aspects of their lives, and less so in others. Although there are individual traits that enhance resilience, the ability to draw support from social networks and resources plays an important role. In other words, some people have more access to supportive communities or access to people or things that can support resilience. I am reluctant to call this a privilege, though, as it may be that perhaps you have the support of a community that has survived similar adversity for an extended period and therefore has been forced to develop ways to make sense of, cope with, and live with trauma. This may enhance your personal capacity for resilience, but it feels uncomfortable to call it a privilege. This is also one of the things that can make resilience more broadly an uncomfortable concept. Sometimes it positions some people as 'better able' to cope than others, but the reasons for this are many and are also often born from adversity.

For a period of time, my children were being taught to be 'resilient' in primary school, getting awards or recognition if they didn't ask a teacher for help or get upset if they were hurt. While this was well-intentioned, it reinforces the idea that resilience is a personal experience and it is our individual responsibility to get over bad stuff that happens on our own. This decontextualises resilience. While resilience research has highlighted a number of individual, psychological, environmental, and internal temperament factors that seem to influence people's capacity to cope or bounce back or do ok despite adversity including gratitude, kindness, hope, bravery, mental toughness, zest, emotional regulation, social connectedness, and determination, resilience is also collective and interwoven with a family or community's ability to communicate, problem solve, stay connected, and make meaning of adversity.

While research on resilience initially focused on identifying the qualities of individual children who succeeded as adults in spite of childhood poverty, abuse, or neglect, researchers have now shifted to identifying the types of relationships, environments, and resources that can support children to be resilient in the face of adversity (Morris & Hays-Grudo, 2023). Building on the Adverse Childhood Experiences study, there has been attention drawn to PACEs or Protective and Compensatory Experiences. In the same way that ACEs have a 'dose-effect' (i.e. more ACEs equals more impacts), protective experiences also appear to have cumulatively positive effects.

Box 2.3: Ten childhood protective and compensatory experiences

- Unconditional love from a caregiver
- Having a best friend
- Volunteering in the community
- Being part of a group
- Having a mentor
- A safe home where needs are met
- Quality education
- Having a hobby
- Being physically active
- Having structure, expectations, and routine

From Morris and Hays-Grudo (2023)

However, another key finding across the resilience literature is about luck. A longitudinal body of work on resilience (Werner, 1997) followed a large cohort of kids from birth into adulthood. About 1/3rd of them experienced significant adversity and were considered 'at risk'. Of these 'at risk' kids, about 1/3rd of them had seemed to avoid any adverse outcomes of their 'risk'. That is, they seemed to attain academic and social success or functioning despite their adversity. Werner found that these 'resilient' kids had strong bonds to supportive adults; they also seemed to have some capacity to be independent and positive from a young age, with a sense that they had the power to influence their circumstances. However, Werner also identified that resilience could change over time. These kids were 'lucky' to have access to a supportive parent, teacher, or relative. But some also faced multiple stressors over time which depleted their opportunities for resilience. In this way, it is not that some folks are resilient and some are not, but that it is an ongoing dynamic shuffle. And people have points of overwhelm where it doesn't matter how inherently resilient you are; your capacity to cope gets overwhelmed. Similarly, people can seem to get more resilient over time.

Resilience has a few different parts. There is resilience in why some people are traumatised by events that others are not. Somewhere in that space between 'event' and 'effect', there are other factors at play that are attributable to resilience. Resilience is also present in how people recover from trauma; how they learn and are supported to make sense of trauma and learn to cope with its effects. Keeping in mind the concepts of luck and overwhelm, which mean that sometimes people have less opportunities to do this or may be slammed with bad things that mean they can't. Importantly, people can be both traumatised and resilient at once. To struggle is not the same as not coping. And to do well does not mean they do not struggle.

For each of the ways that trauma can impact people, there are signs of resilience. There are ways our physiology, neurobiology, immune systems, and selves have adapted to thrive despite or because of adversity. This is also resilience. However, in the same way that it is not the responsibility of the person who experiences trauma to not experience trauma, it should not be the responsibility of the person who experiences trauma to be more resilient. Resilience is a social, political, and cultural phenomenon.

References

DeYoung, J. (2015). *Understanding and treating chronic shame: A relational/neurobiological approach*. Routledge/Taylor & Francis Group.

Dorahy, M. J., Corry, M., Shannon, M., Webb, K., McDermott, B., Ryan, M., & Dyer, K. F. W. (2013). Complex trauma and intimate relationships: The impact of shame, guilt and dissociation. *Journal of Affective Disorders*, *147*(1–3), 72–79. https://doi.org/10.1016/j.jad.2012.10.010

Herman, J. (1992). *Trauma and recovery*. Basic Books/Hachette Book Group.

Morris, A. S., & Hays-Grudo, J. (2023). Protective and compensatory childhood experiences and their impact on adult mental health. *World Psychiatry*, *22*(1), 150–151. https://doi.org/10.1002/wps.21042

Schore, A. N. (2002). Dysregulation of the right brain: A fundamental mechanism of traumatic attachment and the psychopathogenesis of posttraumatic stress disorder. *Australian & New Zealand Journal of Psychiatry*, *36*(1), 9–30. https://doi.org/10.1046/j.1440-1614.2002.00996.x

Schore, A. N. (2009). Relational trauma and the developing right brain: An interface of psychoanalytic self psychology and neuroscience. *Annals of the New York Academy of Sciences*, *1159*(1), 189–203. https://doi.org/10.1111/j.1749-6632.2009.04474.x

Werner, E. (1997). Vulnerable but invincible: High-risk children from birth to adulthood. *Acta Paediatrica*, *86*(S422), 103–105. https://doi.org/10.1111/j.1651-2227.1997.tb18356.x

Wille, R. (2014). The shame of existing: An extreme form of shame. *The International Journal of Psychoanalysis*, *95*(4), 695–717. https://doi.org/10.1111/1745-8315.12208

3 The impact of trauma on the brain and body

Trauma can impact the mind, body, and brain. Neurobiological alterations associated with trauma are wide and varied but include alterations in the right brain, the hippocampus, the amygdala, the prefrontal cortex, the hypothalamic–pituitary axis, the concentrations of corticotrophin releasing hormone, and the noradrenergic system. Neuroimaging studies have allowed for greater exploration of how trauma can reduce activity in areas of the brain, including the frontal lobe, anterior cingulate, and thalamic areas, impacting executive function, attention and cognitive, memory, affective, and somatosensory integration (Giotakos, 2020).

Well-recognised pathways between fear, threat, and memory are now understood in the context of synaptic and circuitry coding, and their intersection with hormonal and circadian systems (Maddox et al., 2019). Across neuroscience research, there are ongoing linkages being made between trauma, particularly that which begins in childhood, and dysregulation of the stress response system and cortisol secretion (Womersley et al., 2022). Evidence also links trauma to emotional dysregulation, avoidance, suppression of emotion, and expression of negative emotions in response to stress (Gruhn & Compas, 2020). This is likely due to alterations in the networks of the brain that control emotional modulation, such as the amygdala and prefrontal cortex (Andrewes & Jenkins, 2019). These pathways are also thought to impact autobiographical memory cohesion, flashbacks, and dissociation, and impact parts of the brain that link narrative to events or enable us to concentrate in the present without intrusions from the past or worries about the future.

It can be interesting to think about how trauma impacts the brain, and it is also interesting to link ways that people react and are, with changes to parts of the brain linked to trauma. However, there are also risks of focusing on how trauma changes the brain. Changes in the brain are complex adaptations to support survival. It helps us survive if we can kick on our survival response rapidly or keep it on for sustained periods. It helps us survive to have our memories get warped or to disconnect awareness of periods of time. It helps us survive to stay hyper-alert and not be able to tune out our surroundings. It also helps us survive to feel numb or lack emotion.

Trauma alters the stress response system

Trauma has long been recognised to impact activation and sustenance of the stress response system. Stress responses are commonly known as 'flight, fight or freeze'. These are normal and adaptive responses that assist with survival. They occur automatically. We may instinctively flee or become aggressive when we perceive a threat, often before

DOI: 10.4324/9781003530770-5

we have really thought about whether we should. If the threat feels inescapable, we may freeze. As nurses and midwives, we know of the stress response clinically, but we also know what it feels like ourselves. We can all think of a time when something unexpected and momentarily scary happened to us, even something relatively minor like a car pulling out of a side street without warning or a shadow in the dark of a room, looking like a person. There is a sensation felt in our bodies in these moments. Usually, the response is immediate and out of our conscious control. Our heart might be beating fast, our hands sweaty, and any number of other physical changes, including dilated pupils, pale face, or feeling shaky. These are all 'symptoms' of the body's stress response. Often in the moment, we might not be aware of our movements or body, or we may have a distorted sense of time. These are all parts of the way that our brains attempt to keep us safe. Even when seconds later we realise that we are actually safe, it may take up to 30 minutes to feel totally calm again or for the shaky feeling to go away.

When the stress response system is exposed to sustained or repeated trauma, it can become hyper- or hypo-aroused. That is, people who have adapted to traumatic environments may become highly sensitive to any perceived threat and switch into the automatic response state, when others cannot identify a reason why. Conversely, people may appear able to tolerate sustained danger for extended periods without any apparent response. This is an adaptation to living with sustained threat. Over time, the stress response system may 'adapt' so that it stays 'on' for longer periods without returning to a state of calm or switches 'on' when there is no danger present at all. These are some simple ways that the brain adapts to survive trauma, but they can be problematic in other aspects of people's lives.

Relationship of trauma to health and illness

It is well established that experiences of trauma have an impact on health and well-being across the lifespan. In part, this occurs through alterations in the brain, the stress response system, and immune functioning. Trauma is associated with increased inflammation in the body with numerous impacts on health. There are also other complex ways that trauma impacts health and is implicated in illness. For example, many people with experiences of trauma may feel pain more intensely or may not react to pain in ways we expect and may respond to medications differently also, perhaps due to nervous system hypo- or hyper-arousal, or levels of inflammation and stress hormones.

Trauma can also impact the things we need to stay healthy. Humans are pack animals, which means we mostly need connection to other people to stay well. For many people, trauma impacts their ability to feel safe with others and to seek out and benefit from social supports. This doesn't mean that people will have no connections, but it does mean that people may be more susceptible to retraumatising relationships or may keep their social world small to avoid harm. This can increase loneliness which impacts health.

Trauma can lead to coping strategies that impact health. Obvious ones may be drug use or smoking that people may use to self-medicate trauma symptoms, despite secondary health impacts. However, the original Adverse Childhood Experience (ACE) study came about, as clinicians were treating women for obesity and inadvertently discovering that over half of them reported sexual abuse (Felitti, 2019). Often when they lost significant amounts of weight, other trauma impacts such as nightmares or flashbacks started to cause them more life-interrupting distress. Many disengaged from treatment or rapidly put weight back on to retain a level of coping. Felitti and colleagues realised that in treating what they thought was 'the problem', they were in fact removing a solution to a more distressing problem. Overeating, excessive exercise, or sustained stress may all be forms of coping, and without addressing the trauma they distract from, altering the strategy may have detrimental impacts.

I have seen this clinically in various ways. People who exercise a lot, then get injured and can't exercise and then mental distress overwhelms them. People who lose their jobs and then get lost in overwhelming distress associated with things from the past. I recall one woman I worked with who was in her 50s and incredibly highly functioning. Objectively, she seemed to be incredibly functional; she had a long marriage, grown children, an executive leadership role in a stressful and busy profession, friends, and a paid-off mortgage. What was less apparent was that she had been having a long affair, and when that relationship ended unexpectedly, everything else seemed to unravel. Within a year, she was drinking a lot of alcohol, on extended leave from work, injured from a fall, separated from her husband, and also experiencing intrusive flashbacks of childhood abuse. It was hard to see exactly what was the 'coping strategy' and what was the problem in this situation. She had built herself a life where she felt she had control and she was busy and able to not think about trauma. When one bit went wrong, all of her coping mechanisms started to crumble and she was left deep in a trauma hole. Like an avalanche where one little pebble starts to fall and then slowly gathers pace and destruction. In this example, her coping mechanisms were either well disguised (such as the affair) or socially accepted (such as working a lot or being very busy), and when these were removed, she turned to less accepted ones such as drinking. For other people, the coping strategies that are effective for them in reducing the distress of trauma may be more directly health-impacting, for example, using drugs, smoking, or self-harming.

When working with the woman whose life started to fall apart, it was confronting. She presented in a regressed state, not making much sense when she spoke, strange in her affect, and curled up in her body. When she described the trauma flashbacks she was experiencing, she did so in childlike ways – factual and descriptive, describing situations which were hard to hear and caused her obvious distress. The memories of the abuse were expressed through the lens of a child, frozen in the past and expressed in the words and even voice of a child. She desperately wanted help, but that isn't always the case. Experiences of trauma can impact how safe people feel in interactions, including those with healthcare professionals. People may not reach out for help or may make appointments and then cancel, or turn up and disclose and then not return. Through a trauma lens, it makes sense to recognise that people will have different assumptions of how much trust they can place in individuals, organisations, or services. However, this can lead people to avoid accessing preventative healthcare or early intervention. Many people may avoid doctors, dentists, antenatal care, or hospitals for reasons of mistrust, fear, or shame. People may also delay getting changes in their body investigated to avoid questioning, intrusive investigations, observation, or out of self-blame or shame. This can have significant health consequences.

Trauma is linked to physical illnesses

Trauma that begins in, or occurs in, childhood can be particularly impactful on people's health. The ACEs study identified a strong relationship between the number of ACEs experienced and the presence of disease conditions associated with the leading causes of death in adults (Felitti et al., 1998).

Trauma has been linked to a wide variety of physical health issues. Across numerous studies, clear links have been made between trauma and autoimmune diseases, premature death, cancer, heart disease, endometriosis, obesity, stroke, insomnia, chronic lung disease, and gastrointestinal disorders, to name a few. Human bodies have a variety of interdependent mechanisms in place to prioritise survival in the face of threat; these involve catecholamine, the hypothalamic-pituitary-adrenal axis, and immune responses. When a threat is sustained (or the response in the body is), the sustained or repeated activation of these mechanisms can have health impacts. Trauma also seems to impact neurodegeneration biomarkers implicated in multiple forms of dementia.

The ACE study found that people who experience four or more types of adverse childhood events have higher rates of ischaemic heart disease, cancer, stroke, lung diseases such as chronic bronchitis, emphysema, diabetes, hepatitis, and skeletal fractures (Felitti et al., 1998). These findings have since been confirmed across studies, with dermatological, vascular, obesity, pain, and autoimmune conditions also correlated to trauma. Trauma is also associated with pain; that is, people who have experienced trauma may experience more chronic pain conditions or heightened sensitivity to pain. Tsur and Talmon (2023) refer to this as 'posttraumatic orientation to bodily signals', linked to pain sensitivity, body vigilance, and sensitivity to physical symptoms. Conversely, there are also people who have dissociative capacity and may feel less pain.

Childhood trauma in particular is known to distort perceptions of various bodily signals, including sensitivity, awareness, and interpretation. Trauma is thought to interrupt 'interoceptive processing' (Atanasova et al., 2021). Interoceptive processing is the ability to sense and understand your body's internal state. For example, we sense we are hungry and need to eat, or we sense that our bladder is full, and we need to wee. There are physiologic cues, but there is also a 'sense'. This sense is the interoception. Alongside interoception is proprioception, which refers to our sense of the location and movements of our body parts. Trauma can mess with both of these senses, but usually not all the time, just when we are under interpersonal or psychological stress (and probably need these systems most).

Disrupted interoception can impact healthcare in various ways. People may not seek assistance for pain or discomfort due to a disconnect from the experience or a decreased level of awareness of the severity. People may also struggle to give coherent explanations of experiences. Often when we see a doctor or physiotherapist or nurse, they may ask us questions about our body ('where do you feel that?' or 'what kind of pain is it?' or 'on a scale of 0–10, how bad is it?'); interoception can disrupt our ability to answer these questions. People may give conflicting responses, seem unsure, or alternatively, to manage shame, may give answers they think may be acceptable.

In his book 'The Body Keeps the Score', Van der Kolk (2015) identifies an interesting connection between disrupted interoception and overall vitality or sense of aliveness. He describes working with people who have experienced trauma and can't feel whole areas of their body or can't identify where sensations are located. He observes: 'when our senses become muffled, we no longer feel fully alive' (p. 89) and links this to neuroscience. On fMRI, the parts of the brain that help identify sensations from the body (the insula, the parietal lobes, and the anterior cingulate) also coordinate emotions and aspects of 'self'. So, while brains may have adapted to trauma by numbing parts to reduce terror or visceral feelings, there is a side effect of also feeling less fully alive. One woman I saw clinically described this connection between her body and mind as separated by 'fog'. She could sense her body, it wasn't numb, but the messages weren't clear, and she struggled to make them out, as though she was trying to see them through fog. This can lead some people who have experienced trauma to feel always out of place in the vicinity of others, as though their body is always awkwardly in the wrong place or space, unsure where to put their hands or arms or what to do with their feet. In conversation, they may seem stilted or rehearsed or awkward, likely because they are wrestling to manage a body and self that lacks cohesion or selfhood. Another side effect of this experience is a reduced ability to detect threats but also to detect safety. In our everyday lives, we rely heavily on intuition and the information we receive from our internal and external monitoring systems. When these are immersed in fog, the messages can be less clear, the trust in self can be compromised, and self-knowing interrupted.

The relationship between trauma and inflammation is another growing area of research, although the ideas aren't new. It is thought that trauma, particularly childhood trauma, is linked to increased inflammatory markers in the body. This may be a result of dysregulation of the HPA axis and the sympathetic nervous system. The immune system is known to be involved in threat response, releasing proinflammatory cytokines which help the body heal from wounds and fight infection. Both physical and psychological threats can trigger this inflammatory response, so essentially the body prepares to survive in response to trauma, and when the threat is sustained or repeated, altered levels of inflammation and immune functioning can occur, contributing to higher rates of cardiovascular disease, diabetes, gastrointestinal disorders, and cancer. Trauma is also linked to the development of autoimmune diseases, such as rheumatoid arthritis and lupus.

It is not disputed that trauma can lead to dysregulation of the sympathetic adrenaline-medulla and hypothalamic-pituitary-adrenal axes. Trauma (as a form of toxic stress) can also lead to abnormal circadian secretion rhythms of cortisol, the stress response hormone. Cortisol plays a key role in endocrine regulation and may also be a factor in immune dysfunction. Additionally, glucocorticoid receptor resistance may contribute to chronic systemic inflammation. Chronic systemic inflammation is implicated in conditions like irritable bowel syndrome, rheumatoid arthritis, and psoriasis, all of which occur in higher rates with people who also have experiences of trauma (Sun et al., 2021).

It may also be that trauma and immune diseases share a common genetic basis at the gene expression level. This means that genetic factors play a role in how trauma affects inflammation and overall health. This is not to imply that genetics cause potentially traumatic events, but rather that they may be implicated in how the body responds to these events and inflammation may exist on the same causative pathway. Like the brain, the immune system is not fully formed at birth but develops in response to environmental stimuli. This is presumably an adaptive set-up, to enable infants to maximise adaptation to the individual's unique environment, but may also reflect a need for immune suppression during the birthing process. Like the brain, the immune system plays a role of surveillance and defence and can become hyper aroused in response to stimuli (Danese & J Lewis, 2017). Studies have found that cumulative exposure to childhood trauma is associated with significant and graded elevation in inflammation levels across adulthood, even when accounting for other factors that may confound this. Elevated inflammation levels and impaired immunity are not just related to interpersonal or attachment trauma but also to things like bullying. Alongside these experiences, there are also many less direct ways that trauma may impact health, for example, through impacted sleep. Many people who have experienced trauma have difficulty sleeping, with sleep known to be crucial for health and well-being.

Trauma is linked to mental illnesses

Across decades of research, trauma is recognised as a significant risk factor for mental illness. It can precipitate illness, as well as slow down recovery. In fact, trauma is the most significant risk factor for the development of all the most common diagnoses. Trauma also has a negative effect on the course of illness, including severity and chronicity. The single most significant predictor that an individual will end up in the mental health system is a history of childhood trauma, and the more severe and prolonged the trauma, the more severe the psychological health consequences. Trauma is associated with increased risk of suicide, as well as more severe emotional dysregulation, and is negatively correlated to the course of many illnesses.

Trauma is also correlated to the development of various personality disorders. People who live with personality disorders may access mental healthcare due to emotional dysregulation. It makes sense that trauma impacts personality development and can also play a role in the development of personality disorders. Personality is the outward expression of our 'self' (which is an internal thing). Personality is essentially how our 'self' interacts with the world and others. Our 'self' and our 'personality' can overlap or be dramatically different. That is to say that sometimes people present a version of themselves to the world which is quite different from their internal self. Self develops relationally throughout infancy, childhood, and into adulthood and can be impacted at any stage by trauma, particularly in childhood. When I think about personality disorders, I think about the ways that people have had to develop complex mechanisms and techniques to get their needs met. This is often (but not always) due to the presence of relational trauma during personality development. People with personality disorders have likely developed traits that protect their 'self' and meet their core needs, in a wider environmental and relational context.

Trauma does not always result in mental illness or disorder. There are many factors which may mediate the relationship between trauma and mental illness. Trauma is associated with emotional dysregulation, and this is understood to be a fundamental mechanism of nearly all psychiatric disorders (Schore, 2002). In addition, shame may play a role (Davies et al., 2025). It is also important to know that experiencing mental illness or altered affective or perceptual states can itself be traumatic, as can experiences of enforced or involuntary care. Trauma can thus be woven into the development, experience, and recovery of mental illness.

Trauma can be expressed as a coping strategy

Many of the ways that the body and mind try to cope with exposure to potentially traumatic events are the same things that cause problems, whether that refers to autonomic stress responses, overactive inflammatory mechanisms, or self-soothing behaviours. John Briere talks about *distress reduction behaviours* (Briere, 2019). These are the same behaviours that we might also call 'challenging' or 'maladaptive', for example, aggression, self-harm, eating disturbances, compulsive behaviours, and so on. They can include using substances, self-harming, and engaging in risk-taking behaviours; they may also include things that are framed more positively in society, like training for a marathon, working extra-long days, or cleaning our houses obsessively. These are all things that we might do to reduce distress (keeping in mind that we might also do these things for other reasons!). They may be effective, yet sometimes they cause us problems as well. Many adult coping mechanisms that are displayed at times of stress, distress, pain, uncertainty, fear, or loss of control may be related to strategies developed across the lifespan, to protect during or from adversity, and can be understood as attempts at coping, connecting, or communicating (Sweeney et al., 2018). Viewing experiences and responses in this way shifts our thinking towards a more ecological and humanistic way of understanding and ultimately working with people.

Working in mental health services, engaging with the extremes of what humans can do to themselves is a part of everyday work. For many people, it can be incredibly hard to understand the reasons why people may engage in self-harm or to comprehend the ways that causing immense pain and damage to self could be distress reducing. Yet in mental healthcare, we witness this paradox constantly. People frequently describe escalating self-harm as: a way to release pressure, symbolically represent the pain they already feel, to viscerally punish themselves for shameful experiences, to reduce pain, or as though one part of themselves is giving the other what it perceives it 'deserves'. We work with people who hide their self-harm in shame, and we work with others who seem to want to show it to us as nurses – seeking out the shock in our faces or eliciting some kind of response. Unfortunately, so often, our responses are of shock or violence or shame or containment, and this too becomes part of the distress reducing-creating-reducing-creating cycle.

The experience of trauma, and exposure to potentially traumatic events, is not uncommon. Many people who receive healthcare will have experienced trauma in their lives, regardless of the reason for their interaction with services. However, not everyone will identify as a person who has experienced trauma, nor consider that trauma is related to their health or experiences of illness or injury. However, trauma can complicate people's experiences of health, stress, illness, and treatment. Understanding the broad and diverse impacts of trauma upon people's lives allows for consideration that the majority of children, young people, and adults coming into services may have experienced some form of trauma in their lives and that this may exist alongside, or concurrent to, their symptoms or illness, or complicate the symptoms or experiences that they are presenting with.

References

Andrewes, D. G., & Jenkins, L. M. (2019). The role of the amygdala and the ventromedial prefrontal cortex in emotional regulation: Implications for post-traumatic stress disorder. *Neuropsychology Review, 29*(2), 220–243. https://doi.org/10.1007/s11065-019-09398-4

Atanasova, K., Lotter, T., Reindl, W., & Lis, S. (2021). Multidimensional assessment of interoceptive abilities, emotion processing and the role of early life stress in inflammatory bowel diseases. *Frontiers in Psychiatry, 12*, 680878. https://doi.org/10.3389/fpsyt.2021.680878

Briere, J. (2019). *Treating risky and compulsive behavior in trauma survivors.* The Guilford Press.

Danese, A., & J Lewis, S. (2017). Psychoneuroimmunology of early-life stress: The hidden wounds of childhood trauma? *Neuropsychopharmacology, 42*(1), 99–114. https://doi.org/10.1038/npp.2016.198

Davies, K., Lappin, J. M., Briggs, N., Isobel, S., & Steel, Z. (2025). Does shame mediate the influence of trauma on psychosis? A systematic review and meta-analytic structural equation modelling approach. *Schizophrenia Research, 275*, 87–97. https://doi.org/10.1016/j.schres.2024.12.008

Felitti, V. J. (2019). Origins of the ACE study. *American Journal of Preventive Medicine, 56*(6), 787–789. https://doi.org/10.1016/j.amepre.2019.02.011

Felitti, V. J., Anda, R. F., Nordenberg, D., Williamson, D. F., Spitz, A. M., Edwards, V., Koss, M. P., & Marks, J. S. (1998). Relationship of childhood abuse and household dysfunction to many of the leading causes of death in adults. *American Journal of Preventive Medicine, 14*(4), 245–258. https://doi.org/10.1016/S0749-3797(98)00017-8

Giotakos, O. (2020). Neurobiology of emotional trauma. *Psychiatriki, 31*(2), 162–171. https://doi.org/10.22365/jpsych.2020.312.162

Gruhn, M. A., & Compas, B. E. (2020). Effects of maltreatment on coping and emotion regulation in childhood and adolescence: A meta-analytic review. *Child Abuse & Neglect, 103*, 104446. https://doi.org/10.1016/j.chiabu.2020.104446

Maddox, S. A., Hartmann, J., Ross, R. A., & Ressler, K. J. (2019). Deconstructing the gestalt: Mechanisms of fear, threat, and trauma memory encoding. *Neuron, 102*(1), 60–74. https://doi.org/10.1016/j.neuron.2019.03.017

Schore A. N. (2002). Dysregulation of the right brain: A fundamental mechanism of traumatic attachment and the psychopathogenesis of posttraumatic stress disorder. *The Australian and New Zealand journal of psychiatry, 36*(1), 9–30. https://doi.org/10.1046/j.1440-1614.2002.00996.x

Sun, Y., Qu, Y., & Zhu, J. (2021). The relationship between inflammation and post-traumatic stress disorder. *Frontiers in Psychiatry, 12*, 707543. https://doi.org/10.3389/fpsyt.2021.707543

Sweeney, A., Filson, B., Kennedy, A., Collinson, L., & Gillard, S. (2018). A paradigm shift: Relationships in trauma-informed mental health services. *BJPsych Advances, 24*(5), 319–333. https://doi.org/10.1192/bja.2018.29

Tsur, N., & Talmon, A. (2023). Post-traumatic orientation to bodily signals: A systematic literature review. *Trauma, Violence, & Abuse, 24*(1), 174–188. https://doi.org/10.1177/15248380211025237

Van der Kolk, B. A. (2015). *The body keeps the score: Mind, brain and body in the transformation of trauma.* Penguin Books.

Womersley, J. S., Nothling, J., Toikumo, S., Malan-Müller, S., Van Den Heuvel, L. L., McGregor, N. W., Seedat, S., & Hemmings, S. M. J. (2022). Childhood trauma, the stress response and metabolic syndrome: A focus on DNA methylation. *European Journal of Neuroscience, 55*(9–10), 2253–2296. https://doi.org/10.1111/ejn.15370

4 Trauma as a memory

Trauma, except when events are ongoing, is essentially a memory. But it can be a very problematic and impactful memory. It is a memory or multiple memories that live on in the present, shaping us and our world.

Memory systems are complex. A large body of research suggests that there is a dramatic difference between the ways in which people experience traumatic memories versus other significant events. Memories associated with trauma appear to be either stored and involuntarily activated with vivid detail or stored and voluntarily activated as fragmented, incohesive experiences. Often, trauma memories are stored as sensory fragments, known as implicit memories, and require a narrative framework to be reconstructed to be integrated into the cohesive sense of self.

Memories are stored in different ways, due to complex systems in different parts of the brain. The explicit memory system stores facts and life-stories, as well as language, context, and reason. The implicit memory system holds images, sensations, and emotions, including fear associations (or triggers). Implicit memories are stored in the limbic system, and explicit memories are stored in the cerebral cortex. They can be linked; for example, explicit memories can be used to give meaning to implicit memories. For example, when I smell pancakes, I have a very strong response in my body (implicit memory), and then I remember the story from my childhood of why this is the case (explicit memory). In everyday life, recollections of events are commonly stored in both implicit and explicit memory systems. But when we experience intense fear, our brains flood with stress hormones such as adrenaline and cortisol to facilitate survival. These hormones subdue logical thought, to enable us to react quickly, while also disrupting the brain's ability to store the details of events. This means that emotions and sensations of traumatic events can be stored without language or context, and separate from any explicit memory. This contributes to 'triggering'. Conversely, at times, details of events can be stored, without associated emotions.

This is all a bit complicated and nebulous, but one way to think of this is that memories of traumatic events can be *encapsulated*. They are stored in contained and protected ways which are intended to minimise the distress they cause. I imagine them as locked up in a small box in our minds. As a result, they are not integrated into other memories or understandings, and work is required to keep them protected. For example, we might avoid anything that even slightly reminds us of the trauma and over time we need to add more and more things to the list to ensure we don't accidentally activate them. Because they are encapsulated, they can feel scary to be activated. So, instead of being able to touch them and keep thinking, if a pathway leads us to them, they can be suddenly triggered. The box springs open like a jack-in-the-box and

DOI: 10.4324/9781003530770-6

the memory is suddenly out. This feels different from when a usual memory comes into our mind: Triggering is like something unexpectedly piercing the encapsulation, unleashing the memory.

Ideally, memories are woven into our narratives of our lives; we can think about sad or hard things and that may lead us to also remember happy or funny things at the same time. For example, walking down a street near my house, I pass a café where I had lunch with my friend not long before she died. Thoughts of my friend come into my mind and I think about what it was like when she died, the shock I felt. I am distracted and I feel sad, and the memory is hard. But linked to that memory is how beautiful her funeral was, how much I loved her when she was alive, how much I miss her, that funny thing she said … I am not overwhelmed by the thought of her death because it is linked by neural pathways in my brain to lots of other thoughts about her, and soon I am continuing along the street thinking about something much less emotive.

The 'ideal' outcome for trauma-related memories is not that they disappear or are forgotten or repressed or blocked, and also not that they are stored in secure high-security prisons in our mind. There will always be things we don't want to think about or that make us distressed. We may always avoid places or people that remind us of very hard things. But the memories will be there no matter how much we run, and ideally, they are integrated into our story of our lives, and we are able to touch them in ways that don't feel scary or overwhelming.

Experiencing validation or support after trauma is crucial for integration of memories. Feeling safe enough to retell the story again and again lessens its impact and helps our brains to find ways to fit the story into our wider stories of our lives. This is *integration*. Integration allows for implicit and emotional memories consisting of images, smells, and physical sensations to be linked with explicit memories of facts, language, and events, and for experiences and memories to be stored as part of an overall narrative of self and events in longer-term memory storage. Integration of trauma memories does not require us to talk about all the details or bits of trauma, just what feels important. For some people, there may be no need to talk about it repeatedly, just enough to defuse its power and to link it to other stories, feelings, and ideas.

Box 4.1: Cam and his scooter accident

Consider this story of Cam, who fell off his scooter while working as a delivery driver.

> I'd been riding for years. I'm a confident rider, and for work, I have to know how to weave in amongst traffic. I can usually tell who might pull out from far away; it's an extra sense I have developed of recognising slight movements of cars out of my peripheral vision. I joke that I'm the equivalent of an Uber-Batman. I can sense trouble. But, when I got hit, he just came from nowhere. Next thing I know I was on the road and people were standing over me. There was this incredible noise in my ears so I couldn't hear anything they were saying. That moment is frozen in my mind. I can't piece together how I went from riding to being on the ground. I keep thinking that nothing was different on that day to any other day; there was no warning you know? There was no moment before the moment. Even though my body healed fast, I feel like the accident psychologically paralysed me for most of a year.

Every time I tried to get back on the scooter, I just felt overwhelming fear and had flashes of lying on the ground looking up at those faces. How could I be sure today wasn't the day it would happen again? They say lightning doesn't strike twice but I don't think that applies to Uber riders. We are surrounded by lightning. I didn't ride for ages, I just avoided the scooter altogether, I couldn't even look at it. I also didn't order any deliveries myself because I didn't want to see any other scooter riders.

In Box 4.1, Cam describes the intensity of the memory and flashbacks linked to the 'trigger' of the scooter, where getting on the scooter would facilitate a return of the fear and imagery of the event. He was naturally engaging in avoidance, not intentionally of the scooter but of the memories associated with the scooter. Avoidance of things that are linked to difficult memories is not a 'bad' strategy, but it often ends up impacting functioning. It can impact by stopping people from doing things (in Cam's case, working or getting himself around), but it can also impact by starting to move through life in ways that require you to be vigilant to possible triggers. In this way, fear breeds fear. Fear of the activation of the memories leads to fear of possible things that may activate the memories. For example, Cam was initially avoiding the scooter, and then he was avoiding seeing other scooter riders. It may be that the memory starts to become encapsulated such that the security around the memory gets stronger and stronger, and then he can't be a passenger in a car or walk on the roadside of the footpath. It is our brains trying to protect us, but there are side effects of its operation to keep us safe, and often there are still sneaky pathways into the memory.

It is hard to live life with a memory in your mind that you fear touching. Many approaches to trauma therapy focus on establishing enough safety that trauma memories can be gently touched and linked to other memories. This leads to a slow reduction of the security systems around them. Learning to touch the memory gently isn't about throwing you in the deep end and learning to swim; it's about slowly laying down new neural pathways that attach to the memory and start to link it to other memories. It doesn't always work smoothly, and it needs to be done with support to avoid being swamped with fear, but the idea of graded exposure and other similar interventions is to stop trauma memories from becoming encapsulated and to instead integrate them into the web of everyday events and experiences. This doesn't mean that the memory is gone; you may still feel distressed when you think directly of traumatic events or precipitants, but the memory may no longer pop up as often or intensely.

Proper functioning of the hippocampus is thought to be necessary for memories to be recallable (or explicit). The hippocampus plays a role in the evaluation of seemingly unrelated events, comparing them with previously stored information and determining how we should respond. The hippocampus also plays a role in fear, anxiety, and obsessional thinking. The hippocampus is not fully myelinated until we are about 4 years old, which is probably why we often can't remember much from before this time. Before this time, we are, of course, learning and remembering many procedural things about how to move and act and be, but these memories are stored differently. We are also learning about people, trust, and ourselves which can make it very tricky when trauma gets woven into these memories without words. At all ages, stress can interrupt the hippocampus's activity. Even when under extreme stress, we can still usually remember most things, but there may be gaps in our memory, or memories stored with fragmented emotions or thoughts.

Dissociative amnesia, or not remembering trauma at all, is state-dependent. This means that it is the accessing of the memories that is altered, not the memories themselves. Our brains have stored them away so securely that all the roads to them are closed. Under similar conditions to when they were created, these memories may still be retrieved, meaning we may not remember something until suddenly we do. In the 1930s, Girden and Culler (1937) found that when they drugged animals and conditioned a muscle reflex, the reflex disappeared when the effect of the drug wore off and then reappeared when the animals were drugged again. The animals didn't consciously 'remember', and if they weren't drugged again, they may never have required the memory, but at some level, it was still there. This is similar to trauma.

In response to trauma, some aspects of memory are enhanced, leading to intrusive and vivid memories, while others can be impaired, leading to forgotten chunks, incoherence, or repression. The brain has incredible ways of enabling survival. This can also lead to memories being pushed out of consciousness. For example, if a child is experiencing abuse perpetrated by a caregiver, it is often denied by the perpetrator, minimised, or disbelieved. For the child to consciously accept that it is happening and it is unbearable places them in an incredibly difficult position as they rely on their caregiver for survival. However, if the abuse is blocked from their conscious memory, then they ensure their survival by being able to stay connected to the caregiver. Incredible.

Blocking out memories is one incredible way the brain has of coping with trauma; this is known as 'repressed memories'. Repressed memories are those that are not remembered by a person but may 'resurface' or be triggered later in life. Resistance to memories being forgotten and later remembered has been used for many years to discredit people who have experienced trauma, despite delayed disclosure and amnesia now well understood as normal coping mechanisms for abuse. In her book on betrayal trauma, Freyd (1997) quotes Associate Professor Ross Cheit, who gave a speech in 1994 where he said: 'Long-lost memories of sexual abuse can resurface. I know, because it happened to me. But I also know that I might not have believed that this was possible if it hadn't occurred to me. And that is what makes me nervous'.

Ross makes an important point about human nature. There are many things that we find hard to believe until they happen to us. I have seen this in mental health services where people don't believe depression is a real thing until they are deep in the grips of it; people who think obsessive compulsive disorder means just being very organised and structured, until they watch their family member unable to leave the house in incredible distress. This happens across healthcare too, for example, people who view giving birth as a natural and beautiful process, yet are floored when they find themselves desperately seeking as much intervention as possible. Currently there is a battle going on to get recognition for 'long covid' as a legitimate experience with many people not believing it is real, right up until they or someone they love experiences it.

There are also strong forces at work that contribute to what we believe. Many of us haven't experienced cancer or kidney stones or asthma, but we still believe they are real. Experiences that are doubted are usually things that make people uncomfortable and challenge power in society in some way. Dynamics of trauma are uncomfortable. There are many parts of trauma that we find hard to accept, for example, that people who seem nice or upstanding do horrid things to other people in their private lives. I am always bemused when reporters interview neighbours of people charged with shocking crimes, and they say (some version of) 'they seemed so friendly to me … I can't believe it, this a nice neighbourhood'. As though we can automatically detect 'bad people' or 'good people', or as though friendly people don't do horrible things, or horrid things don't happen in lovely places. It is too shocking for us to accept, so we push it away. We also may find it hard to understand why people don't 'just leave' violent relationships or how people 'let themselves' be raped, until it happens to us or someone we love.

Individually, we perhaps also find it difficult to believe that trauma is such a significant and life-changing thing, and also something we could just 'forget'. But there are many things that we forget, and then when we remember them, the memory is clear. Maybe we bump into someone on the street who we haven't seen or thought of for years, but as soon as we see them, we know who they are and remember a whole lot of scenarios related to them that haven't been necessarily forgotten but also weren't actively remembered. Or we forget where we put our keys, and then later when we find them, it all comes flooding back to us how we had left them in that spot. We had forgotten, right up until something helped us remember. Sometimes when people have kids, they relive parts of their own lives that they haven't remembered, even though they seem significant. Like how their parents punished them, or what happened to them at school, or that nickname they had as a child that they hated.

Memories can often lie just out of reach and not be tuned into. Or they can be carefully locked away to protect us from what they contain. This is not woo woo. There is plenty of research about how this occurs. For example, theories include GABA and glutamate amino acids, which control nerve cell activation or inhibition (Jovasevic et al., 2015). Under usual conditions, these are balanced, but under stress, glutamate surges to help us store memories in ways that are easy to remember and detailed. GABA is a tranquiliser which helps us calm down and sleep. GABA can help us calm down after stress; however, GABA may also play a role in encoding traumatic memories beneath consciousness.

Box 4.2: Repressed memories

This story is of Magda's experience of a repressed memory surfacing:

> The best way I can describe it is that it was just out of view all the time, and then I turned my head and saw it and it was a shock but also not a shock at all. I had a procedure to assess inflammation in my oesophagus, a scope. Something about the sensation and also the helplessness I felt. I just remembered. I remembered the abuse. Clear as day. At first, I wondered if I was just imagining it, but after the initial memory, it was like a door had been opened that I hadn't realised was there and suddenly I could see a whole other part of the house. I remembered all sorts of things then, and really specific details about them. When I told my sister, she was sceptical because I had never mentioned it before. How could you forget that? She asked. The best answer I have is that … I just did. It was like a door was shut on things that were horrid and then that scope nudged the door open and now I can't shut it again.

At first, hidden memories that can't be consciously accessed can be protective, but they can also have effects which are detrimental. They can lead us to hold negative beliefs about ourselves or react to things in ways that feel out of our control. Even if repressed or forgotten memories don't have harmful impacts, there can be trauma associated with the betrayal of discovering that events occurred. For example, consider someone who is drugged and then raped. They may have no memory of the event, but if they later see footage of the rape, they may experience a full trauma response because of the betrayal and horror. The betrayal aspect of trauma can be as significant as fear. Betrayal can relate to a sense that we should have been safe, that we were lied to, that we should have been able to trust the person or situation, or betrayal of basic assumptions of humanity. The betrayal of having discovered that you have been harmed can be as traumatic as having known you were being harmed all along.

In this way, consent and intent are important. As humans, we endorse sedative and anaesthetic processes where potentially horrifying things are done to our bodies in the course of medicine and surgery. These processes are not usually traumatic, although they can be. This is partly to do with expectations: we agree to be operated on, or we understand that it happened to save our lives. We also trust that our bodies will be treated with respect and dignity, even when we are unconscious. If later we found out that we were violated or laughed at or unnecessary actions occurred, this could be a betrayal trauma. Perhaps our bodies store memories of the pain and violation in ways we aren't aware of, but it seems that with enough understanding and care, we can recover from unconscious pain and suffering with minimal impact. We may not recover so easily from finding out about fundamental betrayals of our humanity, regardless of whether we remember them.

Trauma can lead to dissociation

Dissociation serves the purpose of separating the mind from experiences which are not possible to integrate. It is different from memory repression as it occurs in the present and can become a pattern of coping with stress even once it no longer serves its primary function. Dissociation is an experience of altered cognition, awareness, or identity.

When viewed through a trauma lens, dissociation is a neurobiological way of tolerating the unbearable. Dissociation is an incredible survival skill that can be learnt very early in life. For example, very young infants who live with caregivers who are abusive or neglectful show signs of retreating into their own experience, disconnecting from the caregiver and their surroundings. Infants display freeze responses when repeatedly faced with a threat, such as a parent being aggressive (an external threat) or an unmet overwhelming need (an internal threat). Infants may look suddenly blank or passive, reducing their movements and avoiding eye contact or connection. Freeze responses or dissociation have an intended purpose of detaching the mind from the body, as well as detaching from another person or situation in the present moment. Dissociation is thus both internal and relational and can have a considerable effect on the ability to maintain a sense of self and other. Dissociation in children can present differently to adults. At times, it can be quite apparent and less well masked; at other times, it can be more difficult to identify. Children may live in fantasy worlds that blur with reality, engage in extensive pretend play, or just be very quiet and still.

Dissociation is a usual strategy that many people use in different ways. Examples of everyday dissociation include when we are under pressure, we may 'lose' periods of time or memory, be unable to recall something that has happened, or, for example, not be able to recall the journey of driving home – just suddenly being conscious that we are there. Often, we can recall some facts about events (e.g. getting in the car) through explicit memory, but we may have no connection to what we felt or thought or how time passed as we drove. Alternatively, we may really need to urinate in a situation where urinating is not possible, so we may disconnect from the sensation for a period of time, effectively 'turning off' some sensors in our bodies to allow us to function. These experiences are common and usually unrelated to trauma. In a trauma context, sometimes this built-in system disconnects to a greater degree to attempt to protect us from traumatic material, sensations, emotions, or memories that may be overwhelming or inescapable. It is a form of the 'freeze' response activated without conscious thought, to enable survival through discontinuation of experience and memory.

All mammals have a freeze response for when fight or flight will not work, to enable survival. From an evolutionary perspective, dissociation is a desirable skill. If you are out wandering the fields as a prehistoric human and a lion has you trapped, dissociation will help you appear dead and you will also not feel being eaten. In the modern world, the 'lions' that we feel trapped by can take different forms, but our brains still do an amazing job of trying to enable survival. However, people who have learned to cope with trauma by dissociating often continue to do so in response to minor stresses. The continued use of dissociation as a way of coping with stress means that people may struggle to feel connected to the present moment and themselves and may have difficulty functioning.

Traumatic memories can be triggered

It is commonly known that trauma can be *triggered*. The term 'trigger' has been somewhat co-opted to mean having big feelings or responses to things, but in the context of trauma, it refers to a specific process. Triggering refers to something in the present activating a memory from the past, which is then experienced in the present. This usually occurs beneath awareness and without warning. Triggers are subconscious reactions to perceived danger from the past. They occur in the here and now, but their response is not relevant to the present. We respond as though we are back in the moment when traumatic events may have occurred. Perhaps every loud noise is an air raid experienced long after we are safe from war, because in the split second before the pre-frontal cortex allows for rational thought, the amygdala has already sounded the alarm and activated a survival response.

Because memories associated with trauma are stored separately in the brain, when something reminds us of trauma, our brain and body respond as if they were in the moment again. This is in part to do with survival adaptations, in part to do with the warping of time within traumatic memories, and also a result of how trauma can become woven into experiences and memories. The hippocampus again plays some role in this process by blurring experiences from the past with those in the present. The lack of integration of trauma memories may also be important, as when activated by the 'triggering', there is less opportunity to redirect thoughts or responses to other memories or cognitions. In other words, because we shut all the roads into the memory, we also shut all the roads out. This makes it impossible to just distract yourself from a trigger. While many people who have experienced trauma manage to function without trauma impacting their everyday activities, many will also engage in avoidance activities to avoid re-experiencing traumatic responses under stress.

The amygdala is responsible for the fight/flight/freeze/fawn responses that make us ready to react quickly to danger and also sounds the alarm for triggers. The amygdala is the first bit of the brain to perceive danger. It can make immediate decisions and begin a cascade of events involving other brain regions before the cortex (the thinking part of our brain) can override its actions with logic. This means that the amygdala can trigger a full-blown survival response before we have a chance to logically realise it is not needed. The amygdala also plays a role in storing memories. Similar to how Artificial Intelligence produces images based on all the images it has been supplied with, the amygdala decides what a threat is, based on past experiences, instinct, and learnt behaviours. For example, the amygdala may perceive danger associated with a smell if in the past a similar smell occurred in the context of something traumatic happening, even if in the present there is no active threat.

The stress response system can be 'triggered' by sounds, sights, smells, or other senses or situations which are reminiscent of trauma, although identifying specific triggers can sometimes be tricky. If trauma has been inflicted by other people, triggers may include slight changes in facial expressions, tones of voice, or dynamics of power in interactions. It is therefore not always possible to avoid all 'triggers', but it is useful to recognise when people are experiencing an autonomic stress response or altered levels of arousal, and to consider what may have led to this occurring.

Our brains are filled with neural pathways. Some pathways are more 'hardwired' than others. For example, I can remember all of the words to a song from childhood and sing them after hearing the first notes of the tune, even though I haven't heard it for 30 years, and yet I struggle to remember my work phone number even though I use it daily. Sometimes neural pathways are linked to each other in more complex ways. We can smell the shampoo our grandparents used and be taken right back to childhood. We may be unable to eat food that we ate once when we were sick. We can hear a song that throws us right back into the memory of an old lover. Sometimes the link is something we are conscious of, and other times things have an emotional impact upon us, and it can take us a while to figure out why. For example, we might react strongly to a situation but can only later realise that it was because a person reminded us of someone from the past, or because someone said some words which resonated with a past interaction. Everybody has triggers. They play an important role in making past memories retrievable. However, in the context of trauma, triggers refer to any interaction, sensation, word, action, smell, sound, song, visual, or experience that activates a neural pathway that leads to the locked box of trauma. Sometimes this results in an intrusive memory or a flashback to a trauma; other times it takes the form of a disproportionate response to something in the present, due to activation of something from the past.

Flashbacks and involuntary triggering of trauma memories are disorienting and scary experiences. Unlike the original experience of trauma, flashbacks may have no clear beginning or end and can feel like they occur without warning. Subsequently, people may organise their lives around trying to avoid flashbacks or triggers. Trying to constantly respond to, mitigate against, and manage intrusive images and experiences from the past can be exhausting and lead to a loss of enjoyment of other experiences. The stress hormones of trauma memories being activated can also interrupt everyday life. Seemingly irrational responses to everyday noises, occurrences, or interactions can also lead people to feel overwhelming shame. Working to regain some control over internal cognitions, responses, emotions, and sensations, while rebuilding linearity between past and present, is a key goal of many trauma-focused therapies.

Box 4.3: The impacts of triggers on everyday life

Consider how these triggers may impact people's daily lives:

Tom was in prison in a third world country as a young man. He is triggered by being in spaces with no windows. This has impacted his work possibilities and stopped him from seeking medical care for minor or major ailments.

Frances was bullied at school. He is triggered by the sound of children laughing. He avoids catching trains during the mornings and afternoons when school children are around and prefers to walk along quiet streets.

As a child, Julia survived a house fire where somebody died. She is triggered when she smells any cooking meat. She is careful about any social event where there may be cooking, and she avoids parks, beaches, and festivals.

Sam experienced child sexual abuse in the nighttime. She is triggered by the dark. She has difficulty sleeping most nights, experiences shame in relationships, and avoids any overnight trip with friends or family.

Leonie was in a violent relationship for many years. She is triggered by any interpersonal situation where there is a power differential. This makes it difficult for her to attend service centres where she has to wait or follow directions, meaning she can't seek support with finances, healthcare, or register her car.

Priya was in a car accident where a passenger died. She is triggered by hearing a specific pop song that was playing before the crash. She avoids shopping centres, events, and weddings and never listens to the radio to avoid unexpectedly hearing this song.

Memories of trauma are stored differently in our brains. They may be stored in fragments, or sensory or emotional ways, disconnected from conscious thought or meaning making. They can become 'encapsulated' and not woven into our other neural pathways and stories; this can lead them to be able to be triggered. Triggering of memories leads to flooding of the emotions, sensations, or thoughts associated with the trauma, in the present. Trauma memories can also be repressed or dissociated from; these are all ways the brain is set up to enable survival. The ideal outcome for trauma-related memories is that they are stored in ways that can be remembered, thought about, and managed. There will always be things we don't want to think about or that make us distressed, but it is less life-interrupting if we can integrate even the difficult memories into the story of our lives in ways that are manageable, cohesive, and make sense to us.

References

Freyd, J. J. (1997). *Betrayal trauma: The logic of forgetting childhood abuse*. Harvard University Press.

Girden, E., & Culler, E. (1937). Conditioned responses in curarized striate muscle in dogs. *Journal of Comparative Psychology, 23*(2), 261–274. https://doi.org/10.1037/h0058634

Jovasevic, V., Corcoran, K. A., Leaderbrand, K., Yamawaki, N., Guedea, A. L., Chen, H. J., Shepherd, G. M. G., & Radulovic, J. (2015). GABAergic mechanisms regulated by miR-33 encode state-dependent fear. *Nature Neuroscience, 18*(9), 1265–1271. https://doi.org/10.1038/nn.4084

5   Trauma diagnoses, treatment, and recovery

There are different ways to understand trauma. The medical approach is just one way. As most nurses and midwives work in medical systems, it seems important to detail the diagnostics of trauma, including how these diagnoses can help and limit people's understandings of themselves and their experiences. While many people are affected by trauma, not everyone will develop a 'disorder'. Disorders are characterised by the impact of symptoms or experiences upon functioning.

Trauma-related diagnoses can assist people to receive appropriate care or treatment, enable understanding of experiences, and reduce inaccurate labelling, but they can also medicalise experiences which are often social, political, and entwined in people's lives. Diagnosis can risk reinforcing that there is something 'wrong' with the person, rather than acknowledging trauma as a response to experiences and events. Diagnoses hold power. They control how professionals talk to each other about patients, how patients are viewed by those providing care, and how individuals present themselves to society. While many people find trauma diagnoses individually or practically useful to frame experiences or allow access to services, diagnostic systems can also marginalise and maintain oppressive discourses of what is 'normal' or 'abnormal'.

Post-traumatic stress disorder is one way trauma can present

One possible way that trauma can impact people is Post-Traumatic Stress Disorder (PTSD). PTSD refers to a set of symptoms that occur in the aftermath of trauma. Why some people develop PTSD is not known. Across studies, it is suggested that between 5% and 30% of people exposed to potentially traumatic events will develop PTSD. Risk factors include a history of prior trauma, compounding socio-economic disadvantage, a lack of social support, intentional rather than accidental events, and increased duration of exposure. Things that happen during and soon after events are crucial. This links to the 'experience' of trauma rather than events themselves.

The clinical presentation of people experiencing PTSD can vary drastically. The symptom profile for the diagnosis in the current and fifth formulation of the Diagnostic and Statistical Manual of Psychiatric Disorders (DSM-5), published in 2013 (American Psychiatric Association, 2013), has 20 symptoms, 4 symptom clusters, and a subtype for dissociation.

DOI: 10.4324/9781003530770-7

People experiencing PTSD may present with predominantly fear-based symptoms such as flashbacks or avoidance; or negative thoughts about themselves and the events; or withdrawal and detachment or irritability and anger. Flashbacks, nightmares, outbursts, or severe avoidance are common. PTSD can result in people having psychological and physical responses to stimuli that include specific reminders of the traumatic event (sounds, images, thoughts), but also in response to unrelated stimuli, such as unexpected noises. Responses include physiological responses such as increased heart rate and raised blood pressure.

The diagnostic criteria for PTSD are the same for anyone over the age of 6 years old and are summarised in Table 5.1. All criteria are required to be present, last for more than one month, and not be attributable to any other cause or condition. For children under the age of 6, the symptoms are the same as for adults but may be expressed differently, for example, children may use repetitive play to re-enact traumatic events as a sign of intrusion, they may have distressing dreams that do not link directly the event or where there is no clear content, or they may show decreased interest in play as a negative cognition. If trauma precedes language development, children may not be able to describe what has happened to them, even once language develops, and information may instead be revealed through non-verbal means such as drawings or play. While children's cohesive narrative of events can be influenced by a number of external factors and their sense of time distorted by age, across studies, children have been shown to be able to recall traumatic events accurately and display behavioural alterations, such as inattention or hyperactivity, to avoid thinking about distressing things. Alongside the specified PTSD symptoms, children may also experience academic and learning difficulties, physical health complaints, and interruptions to development, language, and communication.

When people experience PTSD, the recurrent reliving of traumatic events through flashbacks, memories, or nightmares leads to a constant re-exposure to traumatic events, perpetuating trauma. Where the initial traumatic event likely had a beginning, middle, and end, through the re-experiencing component of PTSD, trauma can become timeless, intruding on the present, distracting from the future, and interfering with containing the past. The uncontained nature of this experience can lead people to develop a wide range of avoidance measures to try to interrupt re-exposure. This takes energy and effort and can also make people distracted, tired, and withdrawn or lacking in vitality.

Neuroimaging studies have revealed structural and functional differences between the brains of people with PTSD and the brains of people without PTSD, although it is not clear whether these changes contribute to, or result from, PTSD. The hippocampi of people with PTSD appear to commonly be reduced in size, leading to difficulties in separating the past from the present and interpreting cues from surroundings. In people with PTSD, the amygdala appears hyper-aroused and more sensitive to cues of danger, leading to a heightened 'fight or flight' response, while the prefrontal cortex appears smaller and subsequently is less able to regulate the amygdala's survival response. This means that people may be more sensitive to perceived threats in their current environment, with reduced capability to distinguish the (safe) present from the (unsafe) past and kick into a survival response without time to process their reaction or consider alternatives. In addition, lower levels of cortisol and altered neurotransmitters and hormones facilitate a sustained stress response with delayed return to homeostasis.

Table 5.1 Diagnostic criteria of PTSD

Criterion A: the person needs to have been exposed to actual or threatened death, serious injury, or sexual violence, either directly, through witnessing it occur to others, learning of it happening to someone close to them, or repeated or extreme exposure to details of such events

Criterion B: the person has one or more intrusion symptoms associated with the event (this includes seeing the scenes, hearing the sounds, or experiencing smells associated with traumatic events)	• Recurrent intrusive memories of the event • Recurrent distressing dreams related to the event • Flashbacks where it feels like the event is recurring • Intense or prolonged distress at exposure to internal or external cues that symbolise the event • Physiological reactions to internal or external cues that symbolise the event
Criterion C: the person avoids stimuli associated with the event, including thoughts and memories, people who could resemble the perpetrator, and places or times of day that are associated with where, when, or how traumatic events occurred	• Avoidance of memories, thoughts, or feelings associated with the event • Avoidance of external reminders (e.g. people, places, activities, objects) that arouse these memories, thoughts, or feelings
Criterion D: the person has negative cognitions or moods associated with the event, such as anxiety, sadness, guilt, negative perceptions of self, and a mistrust of the world. This might include an inability to experience positive emotions or a sense of being bad or inherently damaged	Inability to remember an aspect of the event • Persistent beliefs about self, other, or world, e.g. I am bad, no one can be trusted, the world is not safe, I am damaged • Self-blame or external blame due to distorted cognitions about the event • Persistent negative emotional state such as fear, guilt, shame, anger • Markedly diminished interest or participation in significant activities • Feeling of detachment or estrangement from others • Inability to experience positive emotions such as happiness, excitement, love, and satisfaction
Criterion E: the person has marked alterations in arousal and reactivity associated with the event, including being constantly on the lookout for danger, being easily startled or agitated, or difficulties with sleeping	• Irritability or angry outbursts with minimal provocation • Reckless or self-destructive behaviour • Hypervigilance • Exaggerated startle response • Problems with concentration • Sleep disturbance
For the dissociative sub-type: *the person also experiences dissociative symptoms*	• *Depersonalisation: persistent or recurrent feelings of being detached from self or body, e.g. altered time, dreamlike state, or sense of unreality* • *Derealisation: persistent or recurrent experiences of unreality of surroundings, e.g. the world feels dreamlike, distorted, or unreal*

Adapted from American Psychiatric Association (2013).

There is a strong evidence base for treating PTSD

Treatment of PTSD aims to help people live in the present, without feeling or behaving according to responses belonging to the past. This requires traumatic experiences to be located in time and place and differentiated from current reality. Hyperarousal, intrusive reliving, numbing, and dissociation are often the symptoms that most impede separating the present from the past.

Currently, the recommended first-line treatments for PTSD are trauma-focused psychological therapies, with pharmacological treatment considered a second-line option for symptom reduction. Medications (primarily antidepressants) are only recommended if a person can't engage in psychological therapy or in other circumstances, such as when a person is experiencing co-occurring conditions. In practice, a combination of medication and psychological therapy is common (Table 5.2).

Treating any form of trauma in children requires relational and family-based approaches. Children are woven into their context and reliant upon the adults in their lives to survive and to help them build a narrative of themselves and the world. This means that, where possible, treatment should also include those adults. Similarly to adults, effective treatments for child and young people trauma include psychological approaches such as cognitive–behavioural treatment strategies, EMDR, and Narrative Therapy. Common elements of any approach include building supportive relationships, distress management strategies, talking about traumatic events and experiences, challenging unhelpful thought patterns, and a focus on building social and familial relationships. Family therapy and attachment-based interventions may also be indicated depending on the trauma context and age of the child or young person.

Table 5.2 Treatments for PTSD

Psychotherapies	There are many different approaches to psychotherapy. Within these, psychotherapies may address trauma in a variety of ways. For example, Cognitive Behavioural Therapy can help people understand and alter their thoughts and reactions to traumatic events, memories, or triggers; Dialectical Behaviour Therapy can help people manage distress and dysregulation associated with trauma; Conversational model and other psychodynamic therapies can help to rebuild relational trust; Narrative therapies can aid in making sense of traumatic events and reduce their emotional impact
Exposure therapy	Exposure therapy involves gradually confronting trauma-related memories, feelings, and situations to reduce their power over time. This helps individuals process and reduce their fear and anxiety
Eye Movement Desensitisation and Reprocessing (EMDR)	EMDR uses guided repetitive eye movements to help process and integrate traumatic memories to reduce distress associated with these memories. It seems to work by altering neural pathways associated with traumatic memories
Pharmacotherapy	Medications such as selective serotonin reuptake inhibitors (SSRIs) like fluoxetine, paroxetine, and sertraline may be prescribed to manage symptoms of PTSD
Psychedelic-assisted therapies	There is some emerging evidence for therapies involving MDMA, Ketamine, and Psilocybin. Usually, the drugs are administered alongside psychotherapies to aid in processing distressing traumatic memories

Sustained or repetitive interpersonal trauma can lead to complex post-traumatic stress disorder

Many people who experience trauma report a range of effects that do not match those of PTSD. Trauma can be woven into people's everyday lives and selves in ways that can be less specific than PTSD. Complex PTSD results from trauma which is prolonged or repetitive and usually interpersonal, for example, torture, slavery, domestic violence, repeated childhood sexual or physical abuse, as opposed to single or accidental events. It is called 'complex' PTSD because the pathways of effect are present in less distinct ways than those that can be linked to a singular or specific traumatic event. The prolonged and repetitive nature of the trauma leads to traumatic effects woven through affective, relational, and core self-components, impacting functioning in a variety of ways. C-PTSD is most strongly correlated with interpersonal childhood trauma.

While C-PTSD is not in the DSM, C-PTSD is in the International Classification of Diseases (ICD-11). C-PTSD in the ICD-11 includes the symptom clusters of PTSD (sense of threat, avoidance, re-experiencing) with the addition of disturbances in affect regulation, negative self-concept, and difficulties in relationships. This means people may have ongoing mood disturbance, feelings of shame, guilt, or worthlessness, as well as difficulties sustaining relationships or feeling close to people. Many of its most impactful consequences are in relational disconnectedness.

Box 5.1: Diagnostic criteria of CPTSD

C-PTSD is characterised by the core symptoms of PTSD. This means all diagnostic requirements for PTSD have been met at some point during the course of the disorder. In addition, C-PTSD is characterised by:

1   Severe and pervasive problems in affect regulation.
2   Persistent beliefs about oneself as diminished, defeated, or worthless, accompanied by deep and pervasive feelings of shame, guilt, or failure related to the traumatic event.
3   Persistent difficulties in sustaining relationships and in feeling close to others. The disturbance causes significant impairment in personal, family, social, educational, occupational, or other important areas of functioning.

Adapted from World Health Organization (2018)

People with C-PTSD experience long-standing challenges in self-organisation. They may experience intense emotions or a numbness or emotions, feel worthless, or believe bad things happen because of something in them, have difficulties trusting people, or miss the 'red flags' and repeatedly enter relationships with problematic dynamics. To meet diagnostic criteria, these experiences all co-occur with symptoms of flashbacks or nightmares, plus avoidance or a sense of threat related to trauma, and impact upon functioning across domains, in sustained patterns over time. It is also important to consider that C-PTSD involves experiences of deep shame and self-blame, overwhelming emotions, and often a variety of interpersonal coping strategies that work to disguise trauma. As people's memories of trauma or narratives of their lives may be disrupted, it can be challenging to recognise C-PTSD. It takes time and safety to be able to accurately assess for C-PTSD. C-PTSD is diagnosed based on symptom profile and a history of prolonged, childhood, or interpersonal trauma.

People with experiences of C-PTSD can find that the diagnosis alleviates feelings of shame and self-blame, connects them to others, and signals that they are a person who has survived struggles in their life. It can also help people access support or services. While trauma cannot be erased, it is possible to recover from C-PTSD. Recovery may mean that memories of trauma are integrated into a person's life story and no longer negatively impact their sense of self, emotions, and relationships to the same degree. It may mean that people have found ways to recognise and manage the effects of C-PTSD in their lives.

Approaches to treatment of complex trauma

Although much of the evidence base for trauma therapies focuses on PTSD, there is also a lot known about the treatment of complex trauma or other forms of trauma. How these treatments are framed is important, and a trauma-informed lens is required even for trauma-specific services. By this I mean people who present with complex trauma-related distress or symptoms may not articulate their experiences as being related to trauma. There is, therefore, a high likelihood of ineffective treatments being issued unless healthcare workers are aware of the possibility of trauma and how it relates to mental and physical health. Asking for and receiving help is often difficult in C-PTSD, raising lots of conflicting feelings for people and requiring attention to safety and trust. Creating a sense of being safe enough and trustworthy is the first and most important step of any treatment for complex trauma.

Complex forms of trauma are addressed in multimodal ways based on the underlying assumption that central to the experience of interpersonal trauma is helplessness, meaninglessness, and disconnection. The recovery and resolution process is therefore based on empowerment and creation of new connections and meaning, commencing with the development of safety (Herman, 1992). A staged process of guided recovery from complex trauma, inclusive of family and connections, is important in guiding the care of any individual who has experienced trauma and through recognising the wider context of relational safety required prior to processing trauma.

Understandings of C-PTSD include recognition that the 'self' has been fragmented by past adversity which has not been well integrated and many therapeutic approaches therefore target aligning conflicting aspects of the self and addressing ways the past intrudes upon the present.

Judith Herman (1992) proposed a three-phase model of recovery from trauma (Box 5.2).

Box 5.2: Herman's (1992) three phases of trauma recovery

Safety and stabilisation: focuses on establishing a secure environment, and fostering resources and supports to support regulation and self-care. This is about actual safety, but it is also about building safety in therapy. It is only once people are relatively safe that they can work through traumatic memories directly and the associated emotions. A sense of safety is required to enable acknowledgement and engagement with traumatic memories. This will be a process of testing out safety until people feel comfortable that it is ok to stay engaged in the process and to release some degree of control and coping.

Processing: involves the processing of traumatic memories, often by undertaking specialised trauma focused therapies. This second stage usually involves talking directly about trauma, processing memories, exploring the impact of trauma, and grieving things that have been lost. Engaging directly with trauma is important to enable a reclamation of control and meaning.

Integration: the focus is on reconnecting with self, identity, and others. This can include building and sustaining supportive relationships, finding meaning or purpose, and making sense of trauma in ways that are part of the self but do not control or dominate it. Finding meaning is crucial to integrating traumatic events and memories into long-term memory and moving towards recovery. Integration is about how memories are stored, but it is also about people being supported to move past numbing or emotional disconnection and being able to try to connect to others in ways that feel safe and fulfilling.

There are numerous other trauma–related disorders

Aside from PTSD or C-PTSD, people may be diagnosed with other disorders which are linked to trauma, for example, Dissociative Identity Disorder (DID) or Borderline Personality Disorder (BPD).

Dissociative identity disorder

DID is characterised by the presence of two or more distinct personality states. People with DID experience feelings of discontinuity of consciousness, identity, emotion, perception, and behaviour, which are often accompanied by recurrent episodes of amnesia (American Psychiatric Association, 2013). DID is a neurodevelopmental pathway that can emerge with persistent childhood trauma which occurs before the age of 5 or 6. The core clinical feature is a disruption to the sense of self. Under ordinary circumstances, children gradually develop a cohesive (singular) sense of self; however, in the context of severe trauma, people with the capacity to dissociate can seemingly create numerous self-states (or personalities), known as 'alters'.

Sometimes alters have distinct personalities, function independently of each other, and 'take control' at different times. Alters may have different ages or be a different gender from the physical body, have different names, or no name, undertake different roles or functions, and have different attitudes and preferences, different memories, as well as different physical functioning, such as eyesight, medication responses, allergies, heart rate, and blood pressure. Approximately half of people with DID have ten alters or fewer, and half have 11 or more, with people commonly discovering more alters during the treatment process. People may also experience PTSD, amnesia, depersonalisation, and derealisation, a fragmented self, and suicidality. Suicidal thoughts can occur due to depersonalisation or in response to feelings of shame, helplessness, and loss of control. Suicidality in DID is complicated by the possibility that only some parts of the person may want to die.

Treatment for DID is usually long-term psychotherapy with a focus on identification of alters and gradual reintegration. Treatment can be slow, as the three-phase model needs to be effectively implemented with each part of the self, working towards a gradual connection between them. Safety throughout the process is also paramount.

Outside of DID, dissociation can be a common experience for people who have experienced trauma. 'Pathological dissociation' is associated with PTSD (especially the dissociative sub-type), C–PTSD (as an associated symptom), and BPD (in extreme states of emotional dysregulation), although the role it plays in these three disorders is varied. For example, in BPD dissociation can be a transient reaction to extreme interpersonal distress, whereas in PTSD it can be a sustained adaptation to fear, usually taking the form of flashbacks, derealisation, or depersonalisation. In C–PTSD, dissociation can be recurrent and severe, at times not directly related to obvious triggers, but may play a role in extreme emotional numbing and relational detachment. The common experience across these manifestations is a state of physical or behavioural disorientation and shutdown that may be the result of the final stage of the stress response when freeze, flight, and fight responses have failed to restore safety and homeostasis.

It is important to reflect on preconceptions when working with people who experience dissociative conditions. Culture can be a significant factor in how dissociation presents. This is in part due to differences in socially acceptable behaviours and ways of being, but also the varying nature of identity itself across cultures. In some cultures, 'self' is constructed as more relational than in others. Western concepts of self emphasise autonomy, whereas dissociative impacts on identity can challenge the notion of identity as fixed, unitary, and autonomous.

Borderline personality disorder

BPD is a disorder that is characterised by emotional instability, difficulties in interpersonal relationships, and distorted self-image. Diagnosis (via the DSM-5) requires five of the following nine criteria to be present:

1   Frantic efforts to avoid real or imagined abandonment.
2   A pattern of unstable and intense interpersonal relationships characterised by alternating between extremes of idealisation and devaluation.
3   Identity disturbance: markedly and persistently unstable self-image or sense of self.
4   Impulsivity in at least two areas that are potentially self-damaging (e.g. spending, sex, substance abuse, reckless driving, binge eating).
5   Recurrent suicidal behaviour, gestures, or threats, or self-mutilating behaviour.
6   Affective instability due to a marked reactivity of mood (e.g. intense episodic dysphoria, irritability, or anxiety usually lasting a few hours and only rarely more than a few days).
7   Chronic feelings of emptiness.
8   Inappropriate, intense anger or difficulty controlling anger (e.g. frequent displays of temper, constant anger, recurrent physical fights).
9   Transient, stress-related paranoid ideation or severe dissociative symptoms.

Across studies, there are high rates of trauma observed in the lives of people who have a diagnosis of BPD, leading to calls to consider whether BPD is a form of complex trauma. The aetiology of BPD is multifactorial, but there is evidence to support the role of early life trauma as an important contributing factor, with up to 85% of people with BPD experiencing childhood trauma (Kulkarni, 2017). However, there are also people with BPD who have no history of childhood trauma.

There are similarities and differences between the clinical presentations of C-PSTD and BPD. Similarities that present clinically include emotional dysregulation, dissociation, relationship instability, deliberate self-harm, rage, and a sustained sense of 'emptiness'. However, there can also be differences in the ways that the affective, self, and relational components present. For example, negative self-perceptions in C-PTSD tend to focus on a sustained sense of guilt, shame, and worthlessness (which remains pretty stable over time), whereas self-perceptions in BPD are commonly more unstable and fragmented, switching between highly positive and highly negative self-perceptions. Emotion dysregulation in C-PTSD often involves difficulty in self-soothing distress and sustained emotional numbing, whereas emotion dysregulation in BPD is more commonly characterised by emotional lability, uncontrolled anger, and profound emotionality. Suicide attempts and self-harm are considered a core feature of BPD in contrast to C-PTSD, where these issues may be less. Relational difficulties are present in both, but in C-PTSD this is usually characterised by avoidance and detachment based on fear, whereas in BPD there may be rapid engagement followed by volatility, hostility, and alternating idealisation and devaluation of relationships.

The distinct aspects of C-PTSD and BPD lead to different treatment considerations. The treatment for BPD focuses on the reduction of life interfering behaviours such as suicidality and self-harm, reducing dependency on others and building an internalised and stable sense of self (Cloitre et al., 2014). Treatment for C-PTSD, however, focuses on increased interpersonal engagement, development of a more positive self-concept, and engagement in the review and meaning of traumatic memories.

Recovery from trauma is broader than treatment approaches

Many people recover from trauma, even complex forms. This doesn't mean they aren't upset or impacted by their experiences, aren't perhaps able to recall them in vivid detail, or don't continue to alter their lives or behaviour to avoid things that remind them of trauma. It just means that it doesn't impact their lives or functioning to the level required to be considered a disorder, and experiences are integrated into an acceptable narrative of their self and their lives.

Once, I heard a woman being interviewed on the radio very soon after losing her house in a wildfire. She said something like: 'some things can be rebuilt but some things can never be replaced'. While she was talking about actual things, like the loss of photographs and sentimental items, her statement had such resonance of trauma. Many parts of the self and safety and connection and coping can be rebuilt after trauma through safety, connection, and meaning making, but some things may never be entirely replaced. Once the mind and body know of horror or fear or betrayal, it is hard to 'not know' any longer. You may learn to live in ways that those experiences do not dominate or impact, but the knowing may remain. Often recovery is about integrating that knowing into your narrative or tapestry of self and your life so that you accept it, perhaps find meaning in it, minimise shame associated with it, and recognise it as something that happened to you, potentially shaped or impacted upon you, but doesn't define you or continue to take away joy, freedom, and meaning from you.

The good news about trauma recovery is that there are many things that help trauma. The bad news is that it can be hard to know what exactly will help who and when. I have read countless memoirs where people seek answers or describe what helped them recover. A lot of the time what helps might be just meeting the right therapist at the right time, or finding stability in loving relationships or roles in their lives. Occasionally, people find things which help immensely suddenly, like an ex-police officer who adopted a rescue dog, and it radically and immediately altered his experiences of PTSD. For some people, their trauma plays out in their sleep through nightmares or insomnia, and this can be immensely debilitating. But this also means that if you can fix the sleep issue, perhaps you can reduce the trauma effects. I have seen this happen through medications, alternative therapies, or changes in environment. Occasionally, people have a 'break-through' in understanding. Perhaps they suddenly remember or are reminded of something from the past which helps them make sense of something in the present. I've seen this happen through talking therapies, EMDR, psychedelic therapies, and just a coincidence. For example, I knew of someone who struggled with panic attacks related to water, but they didn't know why. Sometimes, even drinking a glass of water could lead to a state of panic. One day, they bumped into someone from their childhood who recounted a story of a near drowning when they were children where they had promised not to tell the adults. The person had no memory of this incident, but knowing about it profoundly helped her understand her panic.

All attempts to help trauma target similar things – reducing the distressing impacts of symptoms of trauma in the present, trying to make sense of and integrate memories of the triggering events in the past, and drawing links between the two. Having awareness of things helps us, but it can take time to really build awareness around trauma.

Box 5.3: Trauma as a big hole we must navigate around

One way that I think of recovery from trauma is to imagine that perhaps initially we are walking along and we fall into a deep hole. The depths of that hole are the trauma; maybe it is full of pain or fear or anger or distress or confusion. One minute we are walking and the next we are in the hole.

As time goes on, we might fall into the hole often or rarely, but we may have no warning of it. Sometimes the hole is where we expect it to be, and other times it just appears in front of us with no time to avoid it. Over time, awareness can help us gather clues that let us know that the hole is coming. It may still mean we fall in, but maybe we just have a few seconds' awareness of what is happening before it happens. Maybe over time, we come to know where we are likely to find the hole and try to avoid it with or without success. Maybe over time we start to fall more slowly into the hole and understand that we are falling and sometimes even grab the sides to prevent the full fall. Maybe over time we learn to walk around the hole, at least sometimes. This is an analogy for trauma recovery. It makes it sound very slow and it can be. But it can also be fast; we suddenly understand the hole and never walk that way again. Or we carry a ladder and rope with us everywhere we go so we can get out of the hole quickly and it reduces the impact on our lives.

Trauma that we can't make sense of or integrate into our understanding of ourselves and our lives is more likely to cause us problems. 'Make sense of' doesn't mean that we have compassion for why it happened, or we find 'the truth'; it just means that we develop some way to understand what happened and we generate a story of it that is comprehensible to us and that we can weave into our wider life story. And there are many ways to achieve that.

References

American Psychiatric Association. (2013). *Diagnostic and statistical manual of mental disorders* (5th ed.). https://doi.org/10.1176/appi.books.9780890425596

Cloitre, M., Garvert, D. W., Weiss, B., Carlson, E. B., & Bryant, R. A. (2014). Distinguishing PTSD, complex PTSD, and borderline personality disorder: A latent class analysis. *European Journal of Psychotraumatology, 5*(1), 25097. https://doi.org/10.3402/ejpt.v5.25097

Herman, J. (1992). *Trauma and recovery.* Basic Books/Hachette Book Group.

Kulkarni, J. (2017). Complex PTSD – A better description for borderline personality disorder? *Australasian Psychiatry, 25*(4), 333–335. https://doi.org/10.1177/1039856217700284

World Health Organization. (2018). *ICD-11: International classification of diseases (11th revision).* https://icd.who.int/

6 The politics of trauma

Trauma is political. While events that initiate trauma may at times be intentional and at other times random, the impacts are sustained by context. Trauma occurs in the context of factors which enable trauma, create trauma, or perpetuate trauma. These include endorsed or hidden violence, social factors which enhance vulnerability or resilience, patriarchal structures, control and power, vulnerability and oppression, systems and structures that require compliance and regulation, technology, rebellion, and resistance. While some events that cause trauma are obviously linked to political and social systems, for example, violence against people because of their gender or sexuality or violence in custodial settings, all trauma inducing events and contexts are linked to their context.

While much of this book focuses on how anyone can experience trauma, this discourse shouldn't eradicate recognition of the disproportionate impacts of trauma across populations. Systemic inequalities and historical injustices mean that some groups within society are far more likely to be impacted by trauma.

Trauma theory makes the political personal

Fires and floods have dominated the country I live in in the last few years. These seem like external unpreventable events, but they are also linked to climate change, de-funding of public services such as the rural fire service, dismissal of Indigenous knowledge, excessive forestry and destruction of natural environments, interruptions to water systems due to damming and privatisation of services, and so on. This makes them political. Plus, people who are more likely to be harmed by things like fires and floods may live in areas where there is less economic privilege or where there is less oversight of buildings or less accessibility to preventative actions or less capacity to rebuild or have adequate insurance, or perhaps where people are living in unsuitable housing or overcrowding. These factors are also political.

If I get randomly mugged and hurt on my way home at night, it could be seen as a random attack, but again, is there adequate lighting and transport where I live? Did my race, colour, gender, fashion, hairstyle, or age alter my vulnerability? What are the social and political factors that are driving members of the community to violence and theft? What resources are freely available to me to support recovery? While the events are not always political, the disproportionate ways that trauma impacts people are.

Trauma can also be inflicted within state and socially endorsed systems such as schools, hospitals, prisons, the police force, and religious organisations. This is impactful for people who are harmed in places where they should be protected or within the very same systems where they are directed for care and assistance, but it also raises questions of

DOI: 10.4324/9781003530770-8

responsibility. It is conceptually easier to frame the problem as residing within an individual, rather than within our societies. Yet all trauma is political. Talking about trauma is also political; it opens the speaker up to being criticised, discredited, or harmed.

While trauma is a sociopolitical experience for many people, the concept of trauma can reduce this to a pathology within an individual. Consider if you are in a room full of sharp knives sticking out from the walls and you get cut, is the 'problem' the wound you got from the knives, or the fact that the knives exist? Especially if only some people have to go into the room with knives, or the room with knives is set up and maintained by those in power, or everyone outside the room who built the room denies the room exists at all. Trauma as a purely clinical, psychological, or pathological concept risks blaming individuals for experiences which are constructed and maintained at social and political levels.

A less metaphorical example of this is sexual violence. Women (including trans women and girls) across cultures and societies experience consistently higher rates of sexual violence within social contexts that normalise and trivialise male perpetrated sexual violence. Women who report rape have their credibility and character questioned in the legal system and are often blamed for what happened through the dissection of their actions, responses, and wardrobes. Experiences of sexual violence are categorised, either in the court of public opinion or in the court of law, as legitimate, horrifying, and perpetrated by a bad person, or of questionable validity, potentially just a misunderstanding or a mistake made by an overall good person.

Box 6.1: Normalisation of sexual violence

This example is Martine reflecting on her experience of the normalisation of sexual violence:

> A few years ago, I was sexually assaulted by a colleague at work ... The main thing I feel now is anger. Anger that I had been friends with him and thought I could trust him. Anger that he felt entitled to do that. Anger that my life changed, and I had to actively avoid him, while he remained unscathed. Anger that I didn't have the energy to go to the police and have to go through everything I drank and wore and said that night. Anger that I have had to push the event out of my mind because there is no other way for me to deal with it. Anger that this approach to coping means that sometimes now I am not even sure if it happened at all. I learnt a lot of things from how people responded that have impacted me in relation to talking about other experiences of trauma in my life. People I told were shocked. 'He seems like such a nice guy'. 'Are you sure it wasn't a misunderstanding?' 'You did spend a lot of time with him, maybe you gave him the wrong impression?' 'Why were you out drinking with him anyway?' 'Are you sure it was rape?' 'Did you try to stop him?' And so it goes on.

Judith Herman (Herman, 1992) wrote about the politics of trauma and how people's symptoms of trauma may present in individuals, but they also occur in the context of wider political and social contexts. She was largely writing about patriarchal systems that uphold and contribute to violence against women, but it is true of many forms of trauma. Acts of violence get reinforced through wars and political actions and sport, abuse gets covered up by organisations and systems, and people in power perpetrate harm and get away with it. The positioning of trauma in individuals is an easy way to minimise having to engage with things that can make us very uncomfortable. To add to this, people who experience trauma are often discredited or disempowered, bringing their testimony into question.

The history of trauma is chequered

Knowledge of trauma has long existed, although there have been periods of attention and interest, followed by periods of dismissal and avoidance. This is largely not due to disinterest, but disagreement. Theories or understandings of trauma emerge and gain traction and then are dismissed by groups in society who find the implications unacceptable. Thus, accepted understandings of trauma have changed drastically over time in response to social and political issues. What we now know as trauma, and particularly Post-Traumatic Stress Disorder, has been renamed numerous times in the context of war, with each renaming subtly shifting responsibility. After World War I, it was originally named 'shell shock' and thought to be a tiny cerebral haemorrhage caused by explosions. In World War II, the term shell shock was banned in an attempt to control its existence. Soldiers were instead diagnosed with 'exhaustion'. Up until the 1970s, it was presumed that people without known vulnerability could experience traumatic events and associated distress, but would recover without needing any treatment. People with long-term effects of trauma were depicted as either vulnerable, from a family with problems, or receiving secondary gain from being sick. This shifted from the 1970s onward when it was renamed again to 'delayed stress syndrome' and subsequently became a mental health diagnosis. The shuffling of how this experience was understood pushed responsibility and blame away from society or governments and back onto individuals, families, or communities.

Definitions of trauma within a diagnostic frame have continued to alter in key ways over time. For example, events that trigger trauma were originally framed as being extraordinary are now recognised to also be quite ordinary; the subjective experience is now recognised as more important than the objective severity of the precipitant; and where originally events had to be directly experienced, they are now recognised to also impact when experienced indirectly, either through witnessing, hearing about, or reading. Thus, trauma has also shifted from something that only impacts individuals to something that can be collective, cultural, historical, and transgenerational.

Critiques of trauma

Understandings of trauma are not without their critiques. One of the primary critiques of trauma is the tendency to focus on individual pathology, often neglecting the broader political and social contexts in which trauma occurs. By shifting the lens from individual blame to systemic factors, we can better understand the root causes of trauma and advocate for more comprehensive and equitable solutions. Additionally, while knowledge of trauma can help us to recognise impacts and challenges associated with trauma, it is equally important to acknowledge the strengths and resilience that individuals demonstrate in the face of adversity. Somehow, there is a dance that needs to occur to be able to hold the duality of the profound impacts of experiences upon individuals, and recognition of the wider contexts which enable these experiences to occur.

There are many other critiques and identified limitations to understandings of trauma. I will briefly overview some of them now.

Critique: trauma is culture blind

This critique focuses on the individualistic nature of understandings of trauma, but in particular how they reinforce assumptions of white, Western culture. Culture can alter how people respond or cope with traumatic experiences, but culture also affects how trauma is defined, experienced, and given meaning. Culture can also impact how acceptable or comprehensible it is to think of experiences as 'trauma'. Culture shapes how people interpret events and, therefore, how traumatic they may be. Culture may also influence what meaning is attributed to trauma-related experiences and what is acceptable to express.

For example, I live and work in an individualistic western culture where people identify 'their trauma'. But I have a friend who grew up in a very different culture, a culture where family is everything and your needs are less important than the family's collective needs. This is also a culture where there happens to be lots of violence. Social and political violence is normalised, but family violence is also common. My friend respects my interest in trauma, but they are also puzzled by it. My definition of trauma would encompass everyone in their family as well as them, yet none of them would consider it trauma or identify with the term. Trauma is not how they conceptualise their experiences.

There are also plenty of examples of this in the clinical context. I have worked with many families where infants are sent overseas away from their parents for years to be raised by extended family members while parents work and then returned in time for schooling. For me, as a parent, to be separated from my infant for years sounds traumatic, and through an attachment lens, it could be considered a disruption in the attachment relationship at both ends of the journey. But in some cultures, it makes sense. Adults and infants may indeed feel sad, and perhaps the experience changes them in some ways, but it is not considered traumatic. Similarly, when mass trauma events occur, individual models of people being affected or needing to talk about their experiences may not align with community needs or ways of coping.

Trauma diagnoses and their recommended modes of treatment are also highly individual-centric and not particularly relevant or useful to many cultural groups. For collectivist communities, approaches that have arisen historically from the community itself constitute their own inherent modes of addressing trauma.

Critique: it is better to focus on strengths

One criticism of centring ideas of trauma is that it can overshadow recognition of people's resilience and coping. I've met academics and clinicians who have said to me, 'I'm not into trauma, I much prefer to focus on strengths'. This seems to imply that it is a binary. That you can only focus on one side of the binary. But, alongside my interest in trauma, I am also into strengths. However, it is my perception that it is still crucial to acknowledge trauma. Pitting areas of academic research against each other as distinct fields rather than interrelated constructs can be problematic for clinical settings and people's lives, where the distinction may be much less apparent.

Trauma makes people uncomfortable, and there is a natural inclination to try to help people 'get over it' or focus on the positives. We are socialised to try to get people to focus on the positives or at least stop talking about the negatives. I am of the belief that to only focus on strengths is something that only benefits people who haven't experienced trauma. People who live with trauma spend much of their lives hiding trauma or trying to pretend everything is ok. It is crucial to recognise trauma before we can move to strengths. Maybe we all know this experience in a more casual way; if we are distressed about something and someone is trying to cheer us up or solve the problem for us, it can feel invalidating or lonely. It can feel dismissive and as though they want us to 'get over it'. We can find ourselves unable to feel cheered up or to think about ways out of or beyond the present moment. Whereas if someone sits with us in the distress, even for a short period, looks around, notices it, says how hard it looks, and listens, then somehow it can feel different and maybe then we are open to being 'cheered up' or drawn towards solutions.

Part of this critique is also that a focus on trauma as a detrimental process fails to acknowledge the complexity of how experiences change us; sometimes they harm us, but sometimes from harm comes growth, which is confusing. Post-Traumatic Growth is understood as a redefinition of self and what is important in the wake of trauma.

I think of a father I met who worried that his children had been too safe. He talked about his fears that they will lack resilience or capacity to cope as nothing bad has ever happened to them. This perception reinforces a binary where either trauma is harmful or trauma is beneficial, when the reality is more complicated than this. Trauma is harmful, by definition. No person who has experienced trauma would suggest it is something they would want their child to go through. But it can also be true that self-awareness, understanding, and growth can occur as part of adversity. Yet there are also other ways to achieve this than trauma. Toughening up children to enhance resilience brings with it experiences of trauma, the impacts of which can't be dismissed. In response to this father, my response was that the harms of trauma do not make it a good deal in terms of possible resilience and coping that may also occur and that his children who have the privilege of safety will benefit from a secure, safe, and loving childhood, even if it means they have to develop skills of survival and coping later in life, in other ways.

Critique: ideas of trauma need to be decolonised

A number of academics and advocates have described the need to 'decolonise' understandings of trauma. It is not possible in the country I work in, and in many countries around the globe, to talk about trauma and not recognise the traumas that have impacted whole communities such as First Nations peoples.

While not all First Nations people experience individual trauma, or identify with the concept of trauma, social and political contexts amplify structural violence for First Nations peoples. For many First Nations peoples, the effects of historical events, including displacement, colonisation, loss of family, narrative, history, language, land, spirituality, and culture, as well as generations of institutionalisation and abuse, have impacts across generations akin to intergenerational trauma. Many First Nations people across the world continue to experience significant social disadvantage across health, education, poverty, employment, and welfare systems and have little reason to trust mainstream organisations, including health services. Thus, although historical suppression of culture and cultural identities has been recognized by Indigenous peoples as contributing to trauma, the solution is far more complex than acknowledging trauma or instigating restoration of cultural practices. To do so obscures ongoing forms of dispossession and disempowerment that occur at all levels of society and deflects attention from ongoing structural causes of distress. Healing for many First Nations peoples goes well beyond trauma therapy for individual distress.

Part of decolonising understandings of trauma is also about recognising the known culturally protective factors that have enabled First Nations peoples across the world to survive, despite significant and sustained past and present trauma across generations. Some of these protective factors include family cohesion, communication about trauma and engagement with community, as well as the weaving of trauma narratives into movement, song, discourse, and folklore (Atkinson, 2020; Marsh et al., 2015). Yet Indigenous healing approaches and wisdom have been largely excluded from dominant discourses around trauma, further negating power through dismissal of knowledge.

Critique: trauma should be seen as a survival adaptation

There is a critique of the framing of trauma as a deficit or maladaptation. Many of the 'symptoms' of trauma are not random things that overcome people (excluding perhaps intrusive flashbacks or nightmares); they are adaptations that people have developed to survive. They may be protective or defensive actions or forms of hyper- or hypo-arousal. To frame them as something wrong with the person ignores that they have kept the person alive, even if they cause functional challenges in other ways or contexts. Even extreme self-harm behaviours have developed to serve purposes of distraction, soothing, or control. This does not mean that people don't require help or that some of these survival strategies don't require further adaptation. It just means that centralising the problem as 'trauma' can further diminish, disempower, and misrepresent.

There are some groups of people who think focusing on trauma as the problem invalidates its role as a survival adaptation. Perhaps if you *only* think of trauma like this, then this may be true, but perhaps it is also not about absolutes. To focus on resilience without acknowledging adversity would be problematic, and to focus on adversity and not recognise resistance, coping, and resilience would also be problematic.

Vikki Reynolds (2020) suggests that rather than assessing, diagnosing, and treating trauma, we may be better placed to witness acts of resistance. Reynolds describes that medical and psychological definitions of trauma obscure violence and suffering by focusing on 'individual brokenness'. In a focus on trauma, we can lose sight of the complexity of human experiences, which nearly always include acts of resistance alongside trauma. This is not so much about resilience or 'bouncing back' from trauma, but about how people have managed to survive and hold onto their humanity in situations and recognising their responses to abuses of power and oppression. These acts can be small or big, and it is irrelevant whether they were effective or not, but they are part of the story, and to miss them and only focus on the harms risks overly simplifying situations and trapping people into roles as victims. This also links to the need to hold onto the political context of trauma.

Critique: hierarchies of trauma are harmful

There is a bit of a problem in the trauma world in how to define and understand types of trauma, without establishing a hierarchy of trauma. Trauma experiences are complex, confronting, and multifactorial, which makes clear categorisation difficult. But yet we persist. Because having language around experiences is important and understanding the details reduces generalisation and misunderstanding. However, what may be traumatic to one person may not be to another, and so then the question is, who decides what is trauma?

Sometimes I find myself frustrated when I hear people use the term trauma in ways that seem to be wrong. Recently, someone was complaining about their work to me. Objectively, their job looks pretty admirable; they get paid a lot to work remotely. They said facetiously that they were thinking of suing their workplace for PTSD from the workplace culture. I found myself feeling outraged: outraged for all my nursing colleagues who go to work and witness death, pain, and suffering; those who try to save people who die, who get assaulted or hurt; outraged for all the people working in very unsafe workplaces. But how helpful is it ever to compare experiences? If someone tells you that their heartbreak is worse than yours because they were together with their partner longer or the circumstances of the breakup were worse, it doesn't help. Your pain is your pain. Hierarchies of trauma are harmful when they are used to invalidate or question people's experiences. But I also see how there is a need to also recognise experiences which are life-interruptingly horrifying or destructive, and to hold these with even more sensitivity than the everyday traumas of existence. There is a risk in comparing and a risk in not. Trauma is both an accepted part of being alive and too confronting to think of. It is a normal response to abnormal circumstances and can also be an abnormal response to normal circumstances, and in some places and circumstances it can be a normal response to normal circumstances.

Critique: trauma impacts disproportionately

It is a complexity for understanding trauma that it disproportionately impacts groups in society. Structural violence means that there are populations that are much more likely to be harmed. For example, trauma can impact people of any gender. But gender can also play a role in the experience and effects of trauma. I have heard many men who have survived trauma describe feeling emasculated or shamed by the way it has impacted them or by the fact that it happened at all. However, across the globe, women and girls (including trans women) experience interpersonal violence in relationships at much higher rates than men. Currently, one woman a week is killed by her domestic partner in the privileged western country I live in. Women's status in society and the patriarchal structures of many societies mean that they may be more likely to experience trauma and less likely to have that trauma recognised. There are pushes to retain gendered language in areas of trauma work to retain awareness of the wider patriarchal contexts in which experiences like sexual violence or domestic violence occur. However, in doing so, there is also a risk that the trauma experiences of people whose gender doesn't align with a binary model are further invalidated. People of diverse genders or sexualities experience higher rates of trauma than the general population. Some of these trauma experiences relate to gender and sexuality, but many do not. People who identify as part of sexual or gender minority groups have higher rates of lifetime trauma, amplified by experiences of structural oppression in society. Interactions with healthcare can also reinforce heteronormativity through rigid systems and practices.

Of course, people may also be part of multiple minority groups at once which adds to their experiences. I had an incredible friend who had done a lot of thinking and working in this space before she died unexpectedly a few years ago. She was trans, Indigenous, a trauma survivor, and a poet. She spoke about this in a way that just made sense. She would describe that she was all of these things, but on their own she was none of them. They were a part of her wholeness, and trauma was woven into all the parts of her physically, psychologically, spiritually, culturally and emotionally. She believed in storytelling and understanding people in all of their wholeness through the stories they tell about themselves, including all the hard and beautiful bits mixed together. Once I heard her equate this to a vegetable soup … where the addition of one ingredient changes the entire soup, and once it is added, even if you take the chunks out, it can't go back to how it was. I think of her vegetable soup in relation to intersectionality a lot. Her description is not mechanistic; one vulnerability doesn't pile on top of another to make more, but the mixture of multiple parts of our identities makes us who we are. If she had not been trans, or if she hadn't experienced trauma, or if she wasn't Indigenous, she wouldn't have been her same graceful, excellent, complex self.

Another tricky component of recognising the disproportionate impacts of trauma is that very privileged people can also experience significant trauma. I read the autobiography of Prince Harry (Prince Harry, 2023) a couple of years ago and I was struck by his experiences of trauma. He is unquestionably rich, white royalty and has been born into privilege and power, but this hasn't saved him from trauma. His experiences of trauma may seem hard for a person living in poverty or disadvantage, or experiencing trauma and lacking the resources to protect or heal, to accept or empathise with. This is also true of many celebrities who live privileged and idolised lives but suffer. Privilege may protect people from some harms and also increase opportunities to access some forms of support and help after trauma, but it doesn't necessarily make trauma hurt less as the experience of trauma is relative to context. This means that for people born into hardship and suffering, what is considered trauma may have a different threshold than for people who have always been safe and protected and who are then unravelled by an experience. It is therefore not possible to compare the events or the experiences because they occur in a wider context of that person's life.

Critique: if trauma is anything, everyone has trauma

Not everyone is pleased with the broadening of the definition of trauma or a focus on prevalence. McNally (2007, p. 280) states, 'We are all trauma survivors now, or so it seems'.

McNally implies that widening definitions of trauma to account for individual experiences means it is harder to quantify trauma or validate claims of its existence. When the term 'trauma' is used flippantly, or excessively, to describe any distressing event, its capacity to capture the impact of horrifying and disastrous acts and events, and their associated suffering, is diminished. However, the idea that trauma is something people may want to 'qualify' for is also problematic and as nurses and midwives we need to be careful to not position people who identify as people who have experienced trauma as somehow manipulating this status for their own gain.

In the 1990s, Freyd (Freyd, 1997) defined a model describing ways that perpetrators of violence or abuse deflect blame and responsibility for their actions back onto victims. The model is called DARVO, which refers to Deny, Attack, Reverse Victim, and Offender roles. DARVO can occur at an individual or social level and encompasses the denial or minimisation of experiences of trauma, attacks on the credibility of trauma survivors, and a reversal where the perpetrator assumes the role of victim either from other compounding circumstances or as a result of the actions of the victim. It has been a long-standing tactic of perpetrators of trauma to establish contexts where the experiences and claims of people who have experienced trauma are disbelieved, questioned for their credibility, or blamed for their own experiences. DARVO is relevant in understanding why questioning the legitimacy of trauma claims is problematic, but also in recognising how diluting the definition of trauma to be inclusive of all experiences is also a tactic to silence those who have experienced harm. The risk is that if we are all trauma survivors, then no one is.

Critique: privileging trauma ignores intersectionality

Trauma is often just one part of people's lives. Trauma does not occur in a vacuum; it is deeply entwined with the complex web of social identities and systemic structures that shape our lives. Our social identities can be protective against trauma, other times contextual to trauma, and other times causative of trauma. We can't know and categorise how trauma and identity intersect without curiosity and openness. For example, many First Nations people live with trauma which is multigenerational and constantly reproduced and reinvented in various forms. Yet not everyone will be harmed in the same way, and First Nations peoples may also experience other forms of trauma, not just related to their culture, or may also experience compounded harm in care due to culture. It is not possible to assume the relationship of people's social and cultural identities to trauma, but it is important to recognise that they may play a role. Intersectionality refers to recognising how multiple aspects of people's lives can amplify experiences, including those of health, illness, disadvantage, or trauma. This means that something that seems 'not that bad' to one person may be really impactful for someone else whose experiences are entwined with social, political, or personal identities.

Another way to think about this is that a patient may experience high blood pressure, and this is a concern that needs addressing. Another patient may experience diabetes, and this is also a concern that needs addressing. If a patient experiences high blood pressure and has diabetes, then their health outcomes will be different. Both conditions amplify each other, leading to a cycle which can compromise outcomes. We don't just call in the cardiac team to deal with the person's heart, without also consulting with the endocrine team. Suddenly, a multisystemic approach is needed, as separating out the two experiences is not possible. The same could be said of obesity and osteoarthritis. The arthritis may cause pain that worsens the obesity, and obesity may also put stress on the joints that worsens the arthritis. Referring somebody to a support group for people with osteoarthritis will not be helpful, as although the other people in the group have some shared experiences, they may also not understand the additional challenges linked to obesity. Plus, of course, it may be that the person is happy and healthy in their body size regardless of its label, and we need to be careful not to assume they view obesity as a health condition. These examples are analogies for intersectionality and recognising how people's unique combinations of gender, class, sexuality, culture, colour, social positioning, and experiences can impact their experiences, including those of trauma. However, we don't dismiss cardiology for focusing so excessively on the heart or invalidate the role that arthritis may play in someone's experience because it hasn't accounted for other conditions that impact. Trauma is impacted by intersectionality, and it is inherently intersectional. Trauma is interwoven with people's lives, impacted by other experiences, particularly those linked to privilege and power.

Within any well-intentioned effort to define or clarify concepts, there is a risk of harm also occurring. Harm can occur through inclusion, exclusion, oversimplification, and over-complication, focusing on individuals or *not* focusing on individuals. Engaging with criticisms, critiques, and limitations of understandings of trauma does not reduce the legitimacy of the work, and justifying the concept repeatedly is also not necessary to prove a need for trauma informed ways of being. Engaging in thoughtful dialogue about ideas about difficult topics and listening to the voices of people who are most impacted is essential for ensuring that knowledge of trauma is retained over time and not dismissed. Interest in trauma has fluctuated across history and experienced periods of attention followed by silencing and dismissal. It is only through engaging with what the challenges have been and recognising the dynamics of power that influence them that knowledge can be sustained.

References

Atkinson, J. (2020). *Trauma trails: Recreating song lines the transgenerational effects of trauma in Indigenous Australia*. Spinifex.

Freyd, J. J. (1997). Violations of power, adaptive blindness and betrayal trauma theory. *Feminism & Psychology*, 7(1), 22–32. https://doi.org/10.1177/0959353597071004

Herman, J. (1992). *Trauma and recovery*. Basic Books/Hachette Book Group.

Marsh, T. N., Coholic, D., Cote-Meek, S., & Najavits, L. M. (2015). Blending Aboriginal and Western healing methods to treat intergenerational trauma with substance use disorder in Aboriginal peoples who live in Northeastern Ontario, Canada. *Harm Reduction Journal*, 12(1), 14. https://doi.org/10.1186/s12954-015-0046-1

McNally, R. J. (2007). Betrayal trauma theory: A critical appraisal. *Memory*, 15(3), 280–294. https://doi.org/10.1080/09658210701256506

Prince Harry. (2023). *Spare* (First US edition). Random House.

Reynolds, V. (2020). Trauma and resistance: 'Hang time' and other innovative responses to oppression, violence and suffering. *Journal of Family Therapy*, 42(3), 347–364. https://doi.org/10.1111/1467-6427.12293

7 What is trauma informed care?

Trauma informed care (TIC) is a way of delivering care, holding knowledge of trauma in mind. Key things include that trauma is common and impacts people in diverse ways and that trauma disrupts assumptions of safety and trust, influencing how people feel, in their bodies, in interactions, and in institutions. TIC also requires an understanding of the ways that trauma can be caused, perpetuated, or retriggered in healthcare. TIC is not a series of steps; it is a way of thinking and being based on holding this knowledge of trauma in mind while care is designed or delivered.

The history of trauma informed care

TIC began in response to growing recognition of the widespread impact of trauma, and the need for more compassionate and effective approaches to care across health and social services. The term 'trauma informed' was first used by Harris and Fallot in 2001 (Harris & Fallot, 2001), who called for social, behavioural, and mental health services to deliver services in ways informed by trauma theory. They emphasised a paradigm shift towards cultures of care where staff learn new ways to interact with the people who access services, in recognition of the prevalence of past experiences of trauma and violence. They were building on work done by the Substance Abuse and Mental Health Services Administration in the United States, and findings emerging from the Adverse Childhood Experiences study (Felitti et al., 1998). Their ideas were also informed by the work of organisations such as women's refuges, domestic violence and rape crisis care, veterans support services, and the consumer/survivor/ex-patient movement in mental health services. These were (and are) spaces where staff engage with people who have experienced trauma all the time and care has needed to evolve to be sensitive to this, long before the words 'trauma informed care' were used.

Defining trauma informed care

In recent years, much has been written about what TIC is. At the core of all descriptions is a recognition that many people accessing services have experiences of trauma in their lives. Subsequently, TIC is a way of delivering care that is underpinned by this awareness. In its most simple form, this leads on to thinking about how care can be delivered in ways that don't activate past trauma or contribute further to trauma. It can then also lead to thinking about how trauma can intersect with experiences of ill health or injury and how trauma can impact engagement with treatment and recovery. In addition, it can lead to thinking about how trauma may impact staff and the workforce. Ideally, to

DOI: 10.4324/9781003530770-9

be trauma informed is to apply that knowledge of the prevalence, impacts, and intersectional effects of trauma to care, treatment, service design, and systems.

Part of being trauma informed is recognising that trauma is relevant to the present and, by definition, not contained in the past. Subsequently, trauma can be present in the room during healthcare, impacting interactions and therapeutic relationships, as well as experiences of health, illness, treatment, and recovery. At an individual level, this requires healthcare workers to prioritise safety in interactions and care, including through the minimisation of power dynamics, betrayal of trust, or fear. Trauma can make people desperately want care, but simultaneously be terrified of it in equal amounts. This can be confusing unless we understand it and TIC puts the responsibility on us as healthcare workers to manage this dialectic.

Being trauma informed doesn't just change the way interactions occur; it is also a shift in how we understand people, their health, and healthcare needs. At a service level, trauma informed services should deliver care that is sensitive to trauma, while removing barriers for people who have experienced trauma. Service-wide approaches to TIC prioritise safe services that people trust and want to use. In the process, TIC highlights issues of systemic trauma and workforce trauma, and the need to think about how to look after staff and how to ensure systemic sensitivity to trauma. Sometimes TIC gets overly simplified to just being nicer to people or 'basic good practice' (Isobel, 2016). While it can look like these things in its actions, it is instead a reconceptualisation of the experience of being an individual coming into contact with services. TIC requires recognition that healthcare itself can be the cause of trauma, either directly or indirectly.

Trauma can be reactivated in care or caused iatrogenically. Iatrogenic trauma refers to harm that occurs in the course of care, in the same way that people may pick up an iatrogenic infection while in the hospital for another issue. For example, consider Joe, who had a successful triple bypass surgery. While recovering in the ICU, he experienced a delirium. Delirium is not uncommon for people after this surgery and was seen as within the 'normal' range of recovery for the staff. However, for Joe the experience of delirium included beliefs that the nurses in the ICU were trying to kill him. This was terrifying. He was also unsure if his wife was involved. While he ultimately recovered from both the delirium and the bypass, it is the psychological wounds of the fear he felt during the delirium, the fear that his life was at risk in a place he should have felt safe, and the overwhelming sense that he needed to escape but couldn't. It is this that stays with him for months after discharge. This is iatrogenic trauma.

Retraumatisation can also occur. Retraumatisation refers to circumstances which lead a person to re-experience a previously traumatic event. The person may be conscious that this is occurring, or they may unconsciously re-experience the same emotions and thoughts of that event without clearly delineating the past from the present. For example, Lucy delivered her baby via caesarean section in a hospital. As a person who had experienced childhood sexual abuse, Lucy had thought a caesarean may be less triggering for her than a vaginal delivery. However, while her baby was delivered smoothly, the experience of the anaesthetic and the sense of powerlessness and helplessness she felt during the procedure triggered intense memories and flashbacks of childhood sexual abuse. She felt she couldn't move or ask for help or something terrible might happen to her baby. The reenactment of her childhood trauma dynamics retraumatised and destabilised her throughout the postnatal period.

There are many subtle and obvious ways that iatrogenic trauma and retraumatisation can occur within any healthcare encounter. Treatments can be painful, scary, or, at times, delivered with force. Care may involve violating or intrusive examinations, painful procedures, shame about bodily processes or functioning, fear about treatment plans or impacts, rigid enforcing of rules, uncertainty about what is being documented or communicated, unwelcoming or unsafe physical environments, boredom or isolation, lack of control over processes, and a lack of transparency and communication about processes leading to powerlessness and fear. Experiences of illness can also be traumatic due to loss of control, fear of the future, loss of hope, or loss of touch with reality.

TIC requires overt acknowledgement that, despite best intentions, harm can occur in the course of care. Once we understand trauma, we understand that the dynamics of care can replicate power dynamics of trauma experiences and that the delivery of care and treatment can be retraumatising for people who have already experienced trauma in their lives. It is not always possible to remove all aspects of care that may be traumatising or retraumatising, but TIC necessitates acknowledgement of this tension and provides a framework for considering how potentially traumatic practices and approaches can be minimised, talked about, and how safety can be fostered within care. Our roles become active ones of reinstating aspects of interactions and care that counteract these experiences, providing people with positive relational moments and modelling safety, trust, and repair. To be trauma informed within existing services requires us to 'look differently' at the way things are done. This requires acknowledgement, opportunities for reflection, and feedback and consultation. Rather than being one big shift, implementation of TIC in any setting usually requires a number of key focus areas or cumulative shifts to bring environments, interactions, care, and treatment in line with the principles of TIC. What these are will differ for each setting and context.

Knowing that care can cause, activate, or be impacted by trauma means that TIC is relevant to all patients, regardless of whether we are aware of their history. Delivering care in ways that are informed by trauma benefits all patients. It is also important because people may not feel safe to talk about trauma, may not recognise how trauma impacts them, or may actively not want to disclose trauma. People may be in a state of shock or activation when they encounter healthcare, overwhelmed with emotions and thoughts from the past and unable or unwilling to clearly articulate needs in the present. Many responses to trauma are ways that the person has developed to cope with, disguise, or minimise trauma and it is important to respect these.

Often, clinicians think they can spot trauma. Sometimes perhaps we intuitively can … we presume it in the lives of our patients we find most tricky, those who are dysregulated and hard to connect with or obviously have such cumulative hardness across their lives. We presume it in the lives of people who flinch excessively or don't want to be examined. We presume it in the lives of people who keep turning up and don't seem to get what they need. But for everyone that we may presume it for, there are so many other forms of trauma hiding, disguising, being activated in more subtle ways, interfering in our therapeutic rapport in ways that don't make sense. Trauma may be also hiding within us, making us respond disproportionately to some people or situations, leaving us shut down from our work, or 'overreacting' to things outside of work. Being trauma informed isn't about sniffing out trauma like a truffle and then enacting the set tasks. A *trauma lens* is a metaphor for an altered way of thinking for those who were not thinking of trauma before. Looking at care through a trauma lens alters a lot of how we see it. I had a book when I was a kid that came with some special blue and red paper glasses that when you looked at each page, wearing the glasses, you could see things that you couldn't see with your regular eyes. This is how it also feels to look at care through a trauma lens.

Envisioning trauma informed care

Many years ago, I saw author and environmentalist Richard Louv speak at the Sydney Town Hall. In the context of environmental change, he spoke about needing to envision a future we want to be part of. He described how many young people have only heard negative things about the environment and the climate, how it is too late to save it, how the damage is done, and so they feel hopeless. This hopelessness doesn't inspire action or engagement. They may recycle and contribute, but there is no motivation to fight for something. He was talking about nature and the environment, but his message resonated with something else I was struggling with. It made me think about health services and TIC. At the time, we were in the early days of implementing TIC in the hospital I worked in, and the messaging was all about all the things that we do in care that cause harm. We were asking people to change based on criticism of current practice and some theoretical ideas, whereas to get nurses and other staff on board, they needed to envision a future for the service that they want to be a part of, one worth working towards. They needed to know what it would look and feel like to work in a trauma informed service. They needed to imagine how a TIC approach could improve patient experience. I had spent a lot of time thinking and talking about what needed to change but much less time imagining or talking about what it would be like if it did. I now think that imagining this is a powerful exercise and should form part of any implementation attempt (Box 7.1).

Box 7.1: Imagining a trauma informed service

What would it look like to be trauma informed in your service or practice?
What would an ideal trauma informed version of your service feel like?
What would people notice if your service or care were trauma informed?
What would it be like to work in your service or team if it were trauma informed?

I have engaged in this imagining exercise with many people over the years. Patients describe that care would 'feel different' (Isobel et al., 2021). They imagine that staff would have knowledge of trauma and be able to talk to people about their experiences and how these experiences influence their lives. Staff would make active efforts to build trust, create safety, collaborate, and provide consistent care with a diversity of therapeutic approaches. Relationships would be very important; the way staff interact with patients would establish the feeling of being trauma informed, but staff would also be confident and knowledgeable about trauma.

When I was first writing this book, I had dinner with my dear friend Ruah. She asked how it was going, and I told her the usual things I would tell people: that it was a lot of work and it felt like it would never be done and so on. I remember that Ruah told me to imagine what it would feel like when it was finished. That was the most important feeling she told me, and it was essential that I could imagine what it might feel like to keep motivated to get there. At the time, I laughed. Ruah was like that, very spiritual and into other dimensions. I think I made a joke about how relieved and tired I would feel. Ruah died before this book was finished, so I never got the chance to tell her that

I was so wrong! That so many times I thought about how proud I would feel when this book was finished, how happy I would feel to look at it and hold it, how impressed I would feel that I had managed to write it, and that she was right, this was what kept me going in a way that thinking about feelings of relief or exhaustion just didn't. We need to like the idea of what the future holds so we can get on board with making it happen. Thus, imagining what TIC may look like in any context is something that can be figured out over time in the 'doing', but it is also very important to spend time upfront imagining it. This is for motivation, but it is also a way to identify whether everyone involved has the same idea of what TIC is.

Criticisms of trauma informed care

It may seem strange to highlight criticisms and misunderstandings of TIC so early on, but there are many and they are all important to acknowledge. TIC is not one thing; it is a way of delivering care and it requires ongoing reflection. TIC is not the answer to all problems, and it comes with its own challenges. Common criticisms include that there is a disproportionate focus on theory and principles rather than any tangible practice which makes it theoretically good but practically meaningless. It can also be seen as a rebranding of ways of working that have long been known and undertaken in other fields, for example, sexual assault services, Aboriginal-led services, refugee health services, and so on. For example, while the discourse of trauma informed has emerged across healthcare and educational settings in the last 25 years, feminist praxis has informed shelters and crisis services for decades, built on understandings of trauma, advocating for social awareness and rights for people who experience trauma, without naming them 'trauma informed'. Yet much of the literature on trauma informed interventions and models does not reflect feminist understandings and practices, leading to understandable critique of the TIC discourse for borrowing the language and conceptual work of women's movements, without the political analysis.

Alongside these broad criticisms of TIC, there are some which are very applicable to the nursing and midwifery context. For example, I have had people tell me they prefer to work in solution-focused or strengths-based models rather than trauma informed ones. Or 'I prefer to look forward, rather than backwards' as someone said to me once. To be able to 'look forward' without being preoccupied with the past or intruded upon by thoughts or dreams of the past or to not have the past constantly impact their present is not always an option. Trauma is loud and demanding and part of responding to it is enforced by an inability to just look forward. It requires our attention so that we can find ways to look forward. Being trauma informed does not require being stuck in the past, but it does require recognising how trauma can impact upon people's capacity to be present in the moment or to focus on the future. I would also argue that even within strengths-based or solution-focused models, we need to be trauma informed.

Another time, I had a psychiatrist say to me (in criticism of TIC), 'If you break your leg, it doesn't matter to me how you broke it'. I think he was trying to say that his role as a doctor is to treat people for what they present with, and it isn't always our role to have to understand why or how the injury or illness occurred. He treats people's distress (the equivalent of a broken leg) and he understood TIC to be asking him to have an understanding of how this distress may be caused by trauma and then to do something about the trauma. He just wanted to treat the thing he knew. I wondered whether he fundamentally misunderstood TIC. But I also thought about whether we do have a responsibility to know about the ways that people break their legs, particularly if they live with repeated or sustained breaks that don't respond to usual care. What if they have a big hole outside their front door that they fall in whenever they step outside their house, do we have a responsibility to ask about the hole or help them recognise the hole, perhaps to try to help find services that can help them fill the hole, or support them to exit through a different door, or find a way around the hole? Understanding things that impact health and recovery doesn't mean we don't treat their sickness (or broken leg), but trauma informed approaches do require us to wonder what might have happened for this person and how that may contribute to what they are presenting with today.

Alongside legitimate criticisms of TIC, there are also many misunderstandings of what TIC is and means. Some of these relate to misunderstandings of the word trauma, and others include assumptions that TIC implies everyone has trauma, that we are being expected to be trauma therapists, or that trauma is positioned as the most important aspect of all parts of care.

At one stage during a TIC implementation process, staff used to refer to trauma as 'The T word' to reflect their frustration that we were talking so much about trauma and using trauma as a reason to change practice. Change felt scary and trauma became the nemesis. This happens often in society; trauma is uncomfortable and people who have experienced trauma evoke difficult emotions. It is easier sometimes to dismiss the concept than to address the discomfort it raises. Healthcare workers may also normalise, minimise, or dismiss trauma due to a lack of understanding, or misuse the term intentionally as a reassertion of power in the face of uncertainty, or to cope with the difficulties raised by the concept itself.

It is important to understand the varying critiques and misunderstandings as part of any effort towards being actively trauma informed. Reflecting on our own assumptions, positioning, and uncertainty is important. To be trauma informed does not require absolute certainty or zealous faith in the power of informing our care with trauma. But similarly, recognising the limitations of TIC should not stop it from being understood as an important part of nursing and midwifery practice. Engaging with the criticisms of TIC is part of being trustworthy and transparent. I have always found it helpful to listen to the issues people raise and to think about why these exist and what they mean. If we leap to being defensive or certain, then we shut down discomfort, experiences, and potentially the voices of people who have experienced trauma. TIC has enough knowledge and wisdom behind it to be able to be criticised and still be important.

The outcomes of implementing TIC

There is a lot of evidence that supports TIC. However, because understanding trauma is complicated, being informed about trauma is also complicated, and therefore measuring outcomes of becoming trauma informed is also complicated. In my experience, this messiness can be used to discredit the approach. I have worked with executives who want to see 'hard evidence' that TIC is something they should strategically invest in. To me, the evidence of the prevalence and effects of trauma is compelling, alongside public health data about the relationship of trauma to health and illness, and brought to life by the qualitative experiences of people who access healthcare and report iatrogenic trauma or retraumatisation in care. If this is insufficient evidence, then there are numerous studies of staff experiences of TIC training shifting their perspective, or knowledge of trauma improving their experiences of providing care. I think it is also a long-standing form of oppression to discredit things which are hard to prove or objectively measure. To me, being trauma informed makes sense in the same way that greeting people to services with a smile and clear information does, or washing our hands to prevent infection, or installing smoke detectors, or treating people with kindness does.

Because being trauma informed isn't one thing, there isn't one main outcome, so it can be difficult to pinpoint the proof that it works. I have worked in roles before where it was my job to evaluate the structured implementation of TIC, and I would often find myself swamped in data, trawling through all the clinical, workforce, and service data available, trying to figure out what would be a good point of measure to focus on. Along the way, I found interesting things, but not necessarily what you would expect, and most of the data was not clean enough to publish. Coercive care reduced, but with it, staff worries could increase, highlighting how restrictive practices can be used to manage our own anxieties. Staff sick leave decreased, but also some staff left the service leading to higher than usual turnover as staff who didn't want to change or think differently about care left. Staff gained knowledge of trauma from training programmes, but this also raised issues when tensions arose between staff who didn't attend or understand the changes, or when staff challenged management about aspects of services that they now understood to be trauma uniformed. Staff reported feeling optimistic and hopeful about the process but also at times identified ways they were already trauma informed and could feel patronised or offended by the implementation processes. Much more time and energy were required to enhance staff knowledge in ways that were safe and adequately paced, well before actual changes in practice occurred. Even after years of implementation, I wasn't always sure what exactly the changes were that had occurred, and rather than looking at 'TIC' as one thing, I had to pivot to evaluating the parts of the work as discrete things, for example, evaluating collaborative care planning processes, reviews of rules, or individual training initiatives. These showed positive outcomes, but how can you ever really capture what it feels like to feel safe with another human, without a comparison group of those people who otherwise may have disengaged or been misdiagnosed or misunderstood? Requiring a cohesive narrative of how it feels to access care can also go against what is known about trauma and what even asking this question may require in terms of power, stress responses, memory activation, and narrative cohesion.

Knowing what I know about trauma now, I can see that evaluations of structured implementation need to be much longer-term, to capture the milieu, trust, and safety that evolves over time and the changing patterns in engagement and recovery that can only really be shown in context over extended periods. I am also a qualitative researcher, so I am much more interested in how people make sense of and understand care in a trauma informed context than I am in proving outcomes. As part of one implementation, interviews with five nurses who had been involved in implementing TIC for a period of 18 months (Isobel & Edwards, 2017) highlighted how changes occurring in the workplace were both good and bad, that change needs to be slow and positively framed, and that they required clarity, consistency, and clear expectation. They were all hopeful for improved care through a trauma informed lens, and they imagined trauma informed versions of care would 'be better', more consistent, cohesive, and flexible. In another project, people accessing services identified that trauma informed services would 'feel different', that staff would be aware of trauma and able to help people draw links between the past and the present, even if they don't directly talk about trauma, that people would have more opportunities to collaborate in care, that services would demonstrate efforts towards building trust and safety, and that care would be flexible and consistent (Isobel et al., 2021). For me personally, I know that being trauma informed in the ways I deliver my care makes more sense to me and seems to be more effective in engaging with people and delivering interventions in ways that support their well-being.

Across studies and reviews and services, service-wide trauma informed approaches demonstrate better outcomes than 'treatment as usual'. This means they seem to work. The most useful approach, when looking for proof that it works, is to search for studies and reviews relevant to your setting of work. There are new studies coming out all the time and they all use different methods. Outcomes generally include things like enhanced patient experience, patient engagement with care and adherence to treatment, as well as staff retention and satisfaction, alongside reduced coercive care, fewer 'incidents', and less staff sick leave. Staff identify that they are happier working in teams that are working towards being trauma informed and this likely also has benefits for patients. There are some tangible things too; for example, some studies track length of stay or engagement in post-discharge care, or even things like cortisol levels in staff hair. Overall, staff seem to report measurable decreases in stress levels and increased senses of competency, investment, and belonging. Patient and healthcare provider relationships improve, care is more collaborative and flexible, and patients have greater self-agency and motivation.

Patients report an increased sense of safety, better collaboration with staff, and more input into care. Implementing a trauma-informed approach with all patients, regardless of trauma history, seems to result in all patients feeling more respected, in control, and comfortable during healthcare interactions. Implementation is also considered cost-effective.

Justifying the question of 'why' services should be trauma informed also needs to draw on gaps in existing services. What do we know about people not engaging, or not feeling they benefit from services? Or not feeling safe in services? Or high staff turnover or sick leave? What do we know about trauma in the community or populations we serve? What do we know about how our unique area of health links to trauma? Implementing TIC is always about solving problems and gaps in existing ways we do and are, alongside benefiting services. This also requires us to keep in mind that moving towards being trauma informed is an ongoing process of learning and can be a very personal process of adapting how we deliver our individual care, alongside any structured implementation approach.

References

Felitti, V. J., Anda, R. F., Nordenberg, D., Williamson, D. F., Spitz, A. M., Edwards, V., Koss, M. P., & Marks, J. S. (1998). Relationship of childhood abuse and household dysfunction to many of the leading causes of death in adults. *American Journal of Preventive Medicine, 14*(4), 245–258. https://doi.org/10.1016/S0749-3797(98)00017-8

Harris, M., & Fallot, R. D. (2001). Envisioning a trauma-informed service system: A vital paradigm shift. *New Directions for Mental Health Services, 2001*(89), 3–22. https://doi.org/10.1002/yd.23320018903

Isobel, S. (2016). Trauma informed care: A radical shift or basic good practice? *Australasian Psychiatry, 24*(6), 589–591. https://doi.org/10.1177/1039856216657698

Isobel, S., & Edwards, C. (2017). Using trauma informed care as a nursing model of care in an acute inpatient mental health unit: A practice development process. *International Journal of Mental Health Nursing, 26*(1), 88–94. https://doi.org/10.1111/inm.12236

Isobel, S., Wilson, A., Gill, K., & Howe, D. (2021). 'What would a trauma-informed mental health service look like?' Perspectives of people who access services. *International Journal of Mental Health Nursing, 30*(2), 495–505. https://doi.org/10.1111/inm.12813

Part II
The Practice

8 Applying the principles of trauma informed care to practice

There are varying principles of trauma informed care (TIC) reported across resources and literature. Here I am using the five principles defined by Harris and Fallot (2001) as I find them to be broad and inclusive. The principles are safety, choice, collaboration, trustworthiness, and empowerment (see Table 8.1). These can be mistaken for 'nice' words or things that we should all do all the time in health-care, but they are actually a guide for how to enact TIC. They are things taken away in experiences of trauma. Nearly all events or experiences that result in trauma involve people losing a sense of safety, having no power or choice or agency, losing trust in people or things, and having no control over what happens. So, intention-ally enacting these things, or trying to, is an important signal of ways to improve care to be sensitive to trauma.

Safety

Safety refers to physical and psychological safety. Safety is not something we decide is present; it is something we have to work towards, using knowledge of what makes people feel safe and unsafe, as well as by attuning to the current situation. Attuning to the current situation means we pay attention to how safe people seem to feel and we pay attention to what we are doing that may be making people feel more or less safe. There are lots of complexities in what it means to feel safe. We can't assume we are safe – this is an important point of reflection … are we safe? To know this requires transparency,

Table 8.1 Principles of trauma informed care

Principle	Definition
Safety	Safety refers to a dynamic and felt sense of being protected from danger, as well as being heard, respected, and attended to
Choice	Choice refers to being offered clear, well-explained, impactful, and enactable options about the way care is delivered, as well as the types of care or treatment received
Trustworthiness	Trustworthiness refers to being consistent, clear, genuine, open, communicative, and doing what you say you will
Empowerment	Empowerment refers to sharing information, knowledge, and power with people such that they can have increased agency
Collaboration	Collaboration refers to open dialogue about perspectives and opportunities for shared decision-making and care plans

DOI: 10.4324/9781003530770-11

trustworthiness, and sometimes open conversations about the limitations of our knowledge, time, scope, or confidentiality. It also can't be assumed that people feel safe just because we think we are safe or that an absence of obvious danger makes people feel safe. Safe or unsafe are dynamic states that can change due to tiny shifts and can also be two things at once. Maybe you feel unsafe walking down a dark lane at night, but maybe you feel safer if there is someone with you or if you are on the phone. Maybe you feel more unsafe if suddenly there is a rustling noise, but maybe you feel a bit safe again when you realise it was a plastic bag. The same happens with psychological safety. Maybe you feel unsafe when you have to walk into a space you haven't been in before, but maybe you feel safer when you see that the receptionist is smiling. Maybe you feel unsafe again when the receptionist says your name incorrectly or when you notice they wear a uniform that reminds you of someone else you know. Maybe you feel safer when they are kind and tell you where to sit. And so it goes on. It is an ongoing dance of safety that occurs from the first moment we encounter people or services and it requires ongoing vigilance from us as workers.

Encounters where psychological risk is detected, including risk of being judged, shamed, or criticised, elicit the automatic responses of fight, flight, or freeze in the same way that physical dangers do. This means people may have an automatic response to some way that we make them feel unsafe either environmentally or interpersonally. Therefore, psychological safety is an essential factor to be able to engage, communicate, and trust. When we don't feel safe in an interaction or place, we can't really connect or trust. We can still be polite and seem present, but we are not able to engage the parts of our brains required to relax and tell a story of ourselves or connect in meaningful ways with others. When we think of it this way, it becomes essential to healthcare delivery that some attempts are made to build safety in all interactions. This doesn't mean that being entirely and absolutely safe in all the ways is our goal. It does mean that we try to create '"some-safety", "enough-safety" or a "safe-r" conversation and relationship' (Reynolds, 2012, p. 27). This is not a random thing that happens; it requires us to intentionally set up an interaction or space to be comprehensible, predictable, and consistent, even moment to moment.

This is really apparent in the clinical context. Maybe we greet somebody in the waiting area or in a clinical space, and you can usually see their eyes darting, their body tense, they are scanning our faces and stance for who we are, whether we are friendly, whether we bring bad news, and whether we are about to cause them pain, fear, or disappointment. Paying attention to how we are coming across in these first few moments is so important for giving off cues of safety – ensuring our body is relaxed, our face warm and open, our voice calm, and our movements steady and predictable. Usually, then people may settle; there can be a noticeable down-regulation of their nervous system in response to determining we are safe-enough. However, this isn't always the case.

Importantly, people who have experienced trauma may have good reason not to feel safe in interactions with other people or services. The cues may need to be more overt or sustained, or we may need to work harder to ensure we give people the time they need to settle in our presence. Subsequently, it is essential to never assume people feel safe and to demand safety or trust or only remove threats and danger but to consistently and proactively provide cues of safety both environmentally and interpersonally.

Box 8.1: Questions to consider about safety

- How do people enter your service?
- How clear is it what is expected of them upon entry?
- Is the initial space welcoming?
- Who greets people and how?
- Where do assessments or conversations occur?
- Is there privacy?
- What noises or processes may people see or hear?
- Are people's belongings safe?
- Is it clear how to get the staff's attention if required?
- Do staff introduce themselves and their roles?
- Are staff welcoming and acknowledge people's presence?
- Do staff smile, listen, and demonstrate respect?
- Is the purpose of interactions made clear?
- Do staff respond to distress or discomfort in ways that are kind and individualised?
- What symbols of power may be present (e.g. keys, notepads, alarms) and have these been minimised or explained?
- Is information clear about privacy, confidentiality, expectations, and processes?

Interpersonal cues of safety will differ for each person. They may be enhanced by considering the factors in Box 8.2.

Box 8.2: Demonstrating interpersonal safety

- Providing explanations of your role, the purpose of interactions, and the processes of care to minimise uncertainty and fear.
- Validating distress and allowing space for people's own descriptions of their experiences and needs.
- Self-awareness of your tone of voice, facial expressions, and body language, as people who have experienced trauma may be hypervigilant to signs of threat, distraction, or invalidation. Acknowledging limitations of your time or role and being upfront about what is possible.
- Paying attention to people's non-verbal cues to identify how they are responding to discussions and interactions. This may include observing for disengagement, dissociation, or agitation. Framing questions in the context of why information is being collected.
- Alerting people if questions are going to be asked about potentially distressing or intrusive topics.
- Explaining processes, particularly those that people accessing care may not be privy to. For example, explaining who you will share information with, what the process of team discussions about care involves, and asking people what specific information they want highlighted in these settings. It may also

include letting people know how to contact staff or seek help at any time and expectations of contact.

- Safety is also enacted through cultures of workplace communication that allow for staff debriefing after incidents, constructive conversations about care, and responsive mechanisms of feedback.
- Fostering accountability for individual and collegial use of stigmatising language or attitudes in the workplace, even in staff areas and meetings.

In nursing and midwifery, often the most powerful intervention we have is ourselves. Therapeutic presence is one crucial way to enhance a felt sense of safety (Geller, 2013). This requires attention to interpersonal space and self-awareness. Therapeutic presence is a shift in focus from 'doing' to 'being'. It involves availability and openness to patients' experiences, openness to one's own experience in being with patients, and the capacity to respond to the relational space. Therapeutic presence requires us to gesture that we are available to listen, understand, and support people to share their context and experiences, even in brief interactions. This doesn't mean going above and beyond or offering more than is expected of our roles, but it involves being therapeutically present within the processes of the care we deliver. This also requires compassion for learnt mechanisms of survival (no matter how problematic in the present) and support for people to form their own understandings of how the past may link to their present.

Trustworthiness

Trustworthiness refers to being consistent, clear, genuine, open, communicative, and doing what you say you will. People who have experienced trauma have likely learnt not to trust aspects of the world, whether that be environments, individuals, services, systems, or their own capacity to control events. As such, it can't be assumed that people trust nurses and midwives or services, regardless of our good intentions and therapeutic approach. Instead, trustworthiness requires us, as well as the wider services we work within, to actively demonstrate our capacity to be trusted. This occurs through honest communication, clear scope and limitations of care, consistency, respect, and provision of information. When a person repeatedly experiences safe and reliable interactions with other people, it begins to create the conditions under which they can begin to trust. Any interaction with a patient can therefore be an important time to provide clear and transparent information about what will happen and to check if there is anything people want to know or ask (Box 8.3).

Box 8.3: Demonstrating trustworthiness

- Being available and direct.
- Being transparent and honest.
- Acknowledging the aspects of care that you have no control over.
- Using respectful language when talking with and about people who receive care.
- Following through on things that you have said you will do.
- Managing your own boundaries (including by managing your own emotions, 'busyness', and frustrations) and being clear about the scope of your role.

Examples of trustworthiness are woven into interactions when we, as nurses or midwives, let people know what we are going to do and why. This can include letting people know when we will be unavailable and how they can access support if they need it, being clear about what the purpose is of all interventions, communicating openly about what is possible and not possible, as well as being consistent in our ways of being.

Collaboration

Collaboration refers to open conversations about perspectives and opportunities for shared decision-making and care plans. Collaboration requires drawing on a person's natural resilience, strengths, and capacity, including respecting their decisions. Collaboration is linked to power, mutuality, and ensuring not to replicate the dynamics of trauma by removing people's agency.

Collaboration is an ongoing process of care. To be beneficial, collaboration should not be a tokenistic endorsement of care by people receiving it (for example, asking people to agree to care plans they haven't contributed to), nor should it be the development of adjunct personal goals that do not impact the main aspects of treatment. Collaboration needs to be meaningful and actionable (Box 8.4).

Box 8.4: Examples of collaborating

- Checking information with the person it concerns, actively seeking input about what is important to document and communicate.
- Co-developing care plans and goals of care.
- Supporting people to think about how they will talk to important people in their lives about their illness or health experiences.
- Supporting (chosen or other) family engagement in care.
- Collaboration requires trust that may need to be built over time. People who have experienced trauma may be reluctant to collaborate with services and individuals until safety is established, maintained, and tested. Acknowledging this can contribute to validating people's experiences.
- Asking people about how they understand what has happened to them, being curious about their hopes and expectations of services.
- Holding the 'narrative' of people's experiences between interactions to promote consistency and respect for their perspectives and expertise.
- Collaboration may also occur through addressing misattunements or misunderstandings in interactions directly by apologising, checking how people are feeling in interactions, or reflecting on what specific approaches people find beneficial.
- Shared decision-making is an important concept within collaborative care provision.

Collaboration can occur within care-planning but it can also occur within other nursing and midwifery tasks like handover or documentation. For example, we can ask people how they want us to document things, what they think is important for us to hand-over and facilitating opportunities for diverse ways to communicate. Some people may be able to articulate immediately what they need, while others may need some time to think, or opportunities to talk with key people, or may prefer to write down their ideas. Part of collaboration is being flexible enough within our scope of practice that we can accommodate people's needs and their ways of expressing them.

Choice

Choice refers to offering clear, well-explained, impactful, and enactable options about the way care is delivered, as well as the types of care or treatment received. Choice means providing meaningful opportunities for people to have control over things that happen to them. Even when choice is limited by circumstances, opportunities to maximise choice are still present and should be actively sought out. Where possible, people should be given opportunities to develop plans for how they want to receive care and in what settings, what helps them when they feel distressed, and who they want involved in their care. This can occur formally through advanced care planning, safety planning, or collaborative care planning.

Choice also requires identifying where there may be micro-options, even within limitations. For example, this might include offering people a choice of where they want to sit, where you will stand, how you will contact them, the time of day for appointments, or the gender of staff who provide care. Too much choice can be overwhelming, so some guidance on what is possible is helpful, alongside establishing ways for people to end interactions when required. Sometimes it is helpful to ask people if they want to be given choices, or what they want you to decide for them. In this way, they get a choice about choice. There may be times when there realistically is no choice because of how unwell they are, in which case this should be clearly acknowledged, tokenism avoided, and follow-up interactions ensured that enable people opportunities to debrief, ask questions, or make complaints.

Choice can be enacted through transparency of options so that people (both adults and children) are aware of the things that have to happen in service delivery and what is optional. People who have experienced trauma may sometimes be excessively compliant or passive in situations where they feel threatened or they may assume they have no choice. Therefore, it may be necessary to explain that there are things that they don't have to go along with and help them to identify which aspects of care are negotiable. Choice also challenges us to think about our roles as individuals within an organisation or service. For example, it may not be helpful for one person to let people do something under the premise of promoting choice, if that isn't the policy that all other staff are following. This can compromise feelings of psychological safety and trustworthiness of the system for people receiving care and create tension that they then have to manage. If a person has found an experience within a service distressing, we should validate the person's experience and distress. We can then give the person a choice about actions they wish to take, including opportunities to give feedback and contact patient liaison officers or complaints departments (Box 8.5).

Box 8.5: Demonstrating choice

- Let people know what choices they have at all stages of care.
- Consider consistent and accessible choices in the way your care is delivered.
- Acknowledge and communicate even when choice is limited.
- As much as possible, be guided by people's own preferences of how they are spoken about and to, and how they are cared for.
- Guide people in how they can access the mechanism of dispute and complaint.

Empowerment

Empowerment is about power. Empowerment refers to sharing information, knowledge, and power with people such that they can have increased agency. It is the opposite of disempowerment. Empowerment is linked to choice and trustworthiness. While empowerment aims to redistribute power, at times I have seen it misused to be a replication of power where we frame our empowerment as an act of helping – leaving people feeling responsible for their own health or recovery, despite systemic factors contributing to health disparities or treatment inefficacy. I have also heard people dismiss the idea that empowerment is possible at all in health, as no person can give another person power. However, I understand empowerment not to be an act of giving people power or assuming people have power; it is primarily about sharing the power that we have as nurses and midwives.

In healthcare interactions, staff inherently have more power than people accessing care as they have access to information, freedom, resources, and set time frames of presence. Power can therefore be shared by ensuring information is clear and accessible, that the goals of people who access care inform treatment and by vigilance to attitudes, actions, and processes that 'disempower' individuals. Empowerment is linked to advocacy and ensuring the voices of people who have experienced trauma are heard and valued within their own care. It requires us to take people seriously and view them as whole people in the healthcare context and experts of their own bodies. People feel legitimised when they are listened to and considered. Empowerment can also be important in helping advocate for patients and also 'translating' medical jargon to patients and families in ways they can easily understand and apply. Empowerment can also be outwardly demonstrated through small acts such as using people's own words in documentation or handovers and respecting the expertise that people hold about their own lives. Empowerment also involves meaningful and genuine consultation with people who use a service, alongside co-design and avoiding tokenism (Box 8.6).

Box 8.6: Enacting empowerment

- Sharing information and knowledge.
- Listening and being curious.
- Advocating for a person and their perspectives within the wider team, during meetings and conversations about people's care, even if they aren't present themselves.

- For people who have lost power through health or other systems, empowerment may involve collaborative planning for how to regain freedom and rights.
- Clear communication about care and treatment, including when people may seem unable to comprehend it.
- Engaging in advanced care planning by helping people develop plans about their future treatments when they are well and then advocating for these plans to be respected within systems.
- Awareness of power: This includes awareness of the ways that we hold and demonstrate power, for example, through access to confidential information, private conversations, locked areas, keys, and documentation systems. Being aware of these symbols of power doesn't change their existence but may allow for more care in their use to minimise further taking away of power from people who access care.
- Sharing power in care can occur through sharing of knowledge. This can include extending a trauma-informed lens to providing people with information about trauma and its effects that they may then use to better understand themselves.
- Creating the conditions for people to identify their own solutions and make their own decisions, in collaboration with the support network of their choice.
- Recognising acts of resistance.
- Workplace cultures that allow for discussion of the tensions experienced by staff in delivering care and create space for safe expression of differing opinions and debate.
- Empowerment can be enhanced by ensuring people can access peer support and connect with other people with lived experience of trauma, illness, or healthcare.

Peer support, culture and gender, and other principles

There are other principles of TIC sometimes identified beyond these five, which include peer support and consideration of cultural and gender issues. Enabling peer support is a means of supporting all other principles of TIC. Peer support can help to minimise the impacts of power and facilitate connection. Peer support can occur by connecting people with others who have similar experiences to enhance mutuality and connection through local groups or networks, or by engaging members of the peer support workforce or through connecting people to external peer-led organisations and resources. It may take people time to engage with the ideas of trauma. Ensuring people have access to peer support and peer developed resources outside of the context of care can aid them to begin to consider how, and if, trauma is relevant to their lives and experiences. Where formal peer support isn't possible, the principle of peer support can be enacted by 'bringing others' into the interaction by broadly reflecting on the experiences of other people who have experienced trauma and using inclusive language that validates and normalises diverse experiences and coping strategies amongst people who have experienced trauma. Peer support can also involve supporting people who access care to identify existing relationships in their lives that are supportive and beginning to co-develop ways for people to start conversations with their family or friends about their experiences or to better engage these people in their care.

Recognition of culture and gender issues should always be woven into TIC. Cultural safety is more than understanding another person's cultural background; it requires all healthcare workers to reflect on their own cultural identity and to also consider the power dynamics that exist in healthcare services. Cultural safety is not an assumption; it requires openness to difference, curiosity about other people's unique experiences, and recognition that we all bring our own cultural lens to our interactions with other people, including within care provision. In a TIC context, cultural safety also requires recognition of ongoing and historical trauma and structural disadvantage that have occurred for many cultural groups, including refugees, asylum seekers, and Indigenous communities. Not only is trauma more likely to be present in the lives of individuals from these groups but also there may be long-standing mistrust of services and organisations that further impact overall safety. Cultural safety within TIC involves asking people about things that are important for you to know in relation to their care and asking about experiences within their extended family and community that may be impactful, while respecting their ways of interpreting these experiences. Long-standing relationships between culture, gender, sexuality, identity, social status, and trauma can lead to differences in how people understand and respond to their experiences, express emotions, and talk about events. It is important that we remain curious and non-judgemental when observing or talking about responses to trauma. To do this, we need to recognise, acknowledge, and reflect on our own cultural assumptions and expectations. We need to recognise the existing ways that many groups who have experienced multigenerational trauma have developed to cope and build resilience within their cultural context. To be trauma informed requires us to actively seek out knowledge about the wider context of trauma and social responses.

Trauma has historically been, and continues to be, widespread within many identified community groups including people who are gender or sexuality diverse, people from culturally diverse backgrounds, women, and people with disabilities. Not everyone in these groups will have experienced trauma or will conceptualise their experiences through a trauma lens, but it is important for all nurses and midwives to be particularly sensitive to the unique needs of groups and individuals who have experienced cumulative and ongoing invalidation and invisibility within care. It is also worth considering that people may not just have one culture or subculture with which they identify; people may experience intersectional vulnerability or resilience.

Applying the principles in practice

The principles of TIC are all interrelated rather than discrete things. For example, collaborating and providing choice to a person enhances empowerment. Being trustworthy increases safety. Cultural safety is a part of safety. And, so on. Despite how I have laid them out here, the principles are generally intended to guide TIC, rather than be discretely addressed.

When considered on their own, each of the principles can reflect usual 'good practice'. However, rather than being concepts that are unique to TIC, they are guiding principles which assist in delivering TIC, *when they are implemented in a way that is informed by understandings of trauma*. That is, each needs to be considered in relation to each individual person and their context, underpinned by sensitivity to trauma, and universal precautions to reduce iatrogenic harm. For example, it is not enough to try to be safe without considering what might be making people feel less safe, and it is not enough to collaborate in care if we don't consider all the reasons this may be hard (or crucially important) for people.

Having said that, they aren't things that can be discretely addressed. In my own practice, I do think about the principles somewhat systematically in interactions. I might ask myself, 'What could I do to enhance [principle] right now?' I run through the five principles in my head to try to see how I could enhance an interaction; it gives me something to anchor my thinking and it also often directs me on things to do. Finding 'things to do' to be TIC is important, so it remains practical rather than just theoretical. Somehow, running through the principles one at a time can help you reorient to the interaction if you feel stuck, or if you start to feel that TIC is a theory rather than a practice.

Nurses and midwives are under pressure to be person-centred, culturally competent, recovery-oriented, family-focused, strengths-focused, and more. This can make it seem like being 'trauma informed' is just the next thing. All of these approaches draw on ideas of holistic, empathic, and collaborative approaches to care and TIC resonates with each of these approaches; it can underpin them or inform them. But it is also difficult to do any of these without really considering trauma. For example, considering how trauma may be impacting a person and what they need from us in care, recognising how people have developed strengths and understanding these in the context of the purpose they have served in surviving adversity, and also recognising how trauma can emerge from, be enacted within, and impact families and cultural groups. TIC is not a model of care; it is a crucial part of how we understand people and care. To work towards TIC, it is important we imagine what it might look and feel like in practice, while also being conscious of culture and valuing people's own lived expertise.

Reference

Geller, S. M. (2013). Therapeutic presence: An essential way of being. In M. Cooper, P. F. Schmid, M. O'Hara, & A. C. Bohart (Eds.), *The Handbook of person-centred psychotherapy and counselling* (2nd ed.; pp. 209–222). Palgrave.

Harris, M., & Fallot, R. D. (2001). Envisioning a trauma-informed service system: A vital paradigm shift. *New Directions for Mental Health Services, 2001*(89), 3–22. https://doi.org/10.1002/yd.23320018903

Reynolds, V. (2012). An ethical stance for justice-doing in community work and therapy. *Journal of Systemic Therapies, 31*(4), 18–33. https://doi.org/10.1521/jsyt.2012.31.4.18

9 Being trauma informed in interactions

When I was writing this chapter, a friend asked me where I was up to with the book. When I said I was writing about how to have interactions with people who have experienced trauma, my friend said, 'Oh, is there a trick to it?' Their question threw me for a while as I turned it over in my mind – is there a trick to it? Is this just about how we interact with anyone in our roles? Why does it matter if someone has experienced trauma or not? In one way, no, there isn't a trick to it; all our interactions as nurses and midwives should be conducted in ways that foster safety and trust, and it is this that is at the heart of being trauma informed. But in another, yes, there is a trick to it; trauma informed interactions require an intentional use of attention and awareness to monitor relational safety in the moment, in a way that supports people to stay connected. It is a slight shift in a way of being that has profound impacts on people.

The therapeutic relationship is key to all nursing and midwifery practice. Therapeutic relationships require therapeutic presence. Therapeutic presence refers to bringing ourselves to the engagement with the person, being present in the moment, and paying attention to their needs. Therapeutic presence facilitates people feeling safe in any relationship, even brief or clinical ones. Across nursing and midwifery practice, therapeutic presence can be the most beneficial thing we offer patients. Maybe the best way to think about what therapeutic presence is is in our personal lives (Boxes 9.1).

Box 9.1: Therapeutic presence

Consider these scenarios:

Imagine you are going to visit a friend who is sick or going through something big. They are feeling very low and sad, and you pop around to see them. You know they need you and aren't in any place to hold your current news or feelings. No matter what else is going on in your life, you try to centre yourself before entering their space, you clear some space in your busy head and life to really see how they are, to sit and listen and to notice. How do you do this? How do you approach them? What do you say and look for in response? How do you signal to them that you care and are listening?

If you have children or young people in your life, imagine how you manage to stop whatever you are doing to listen to what they are telling you about their day if they are upset or proud or confused about something important. Maybe you are straight in the door from work, but how do you clear your mind and focus on

---

DOI: 10.4324/9781003530770-12

them? What do you pay attention to as they are telling you what happened? How do you signal to them that you care and are listening?

Imagine you are going on a date with someone new, your partner, or even a friend. You had a busy day at work and some difficult things happened, but it feels really important that you put on your best self and pay attention to the person you are on a date with. How do you do this? How do you put aside your work stress and focus on the date? How do you pay attention to them, while also trying to demonstrate how engaged and listening you are, while also keeping track of the wider context of the date and how it's going?

Therapeutic presence exists in the details of how we are with people. What we do with our bodies, our faces, our minds, our voices, our eyes, and our energy. We aren't usually concentrating on these things; we are just doing. But it can be helpful to concentrate on them to identify how we do it, or how other people do it in ways that we like, and therefore how we can improve. Perhaps you know someone in your life who is a good listener or always makes you feel safe. Or perhaps you meet someone momentarily somewhere out in the world or at an event, and you feel that even in a few moments of being with them, they really seem to see you or hear you. How did they do that?

Therapeutic presence requires us to concurrently be grounded within ourselves, be open and receptive to the patient and what is important to them, and also maintain awareness of the situation and surroundings. It's important always in healthcare, but it's crucial for TIC. This has three components – our internal state, our connection to the patient, and our wider context. It is both complex and simple; it is what is happening when we are in the 'flow' of our nursing and midwifery practice and providing care to people in ways that are responsive and sensitive, but it also takes intention and attention. Perhaps we notice most when this doesn't happen; there may be things going on in our own professional or personal lives that interrupt our internal state and capacity to be present. We can be unsettled by a weird interaction that just happened with a colleague (past), worrying about how we will get everything done before handover (future), distracted because we didn't sleep well last night after a disagreement with our flatmate (past), or thinking about whether we have time for lunch (future). There may be patients who we struggle to connect with because of their presentation, personality, culture, or circumstance, but there may also be times when they are shutting us down from connecting to them or we are avoiding connecting to them as we lack time, compassion, or interest. There are also contextual things that impact, maybe we are lacking confidence or new and so we are overly concentrating on what we are doing at the cost of the person, maybe we are distracted by looking at a computer or notes and missing non-verbal cues, or maybe there are other factors or people distracting us.

These things happen all the time in clinical practice and to be trauma informed is not to be immune to this or requiring perfection; it is just about being conscious of it and taking responsibility for trying to correct aspects within our control. We can't make people connect to us or feel safe with us, but we can do lots of things on our side of the equation to make this more likely to occur. And when holding knowledge of trauma, this becomes central to the work that we are doing. If we pay attention and do a few things and they connect easily and things go smoothly, then nothing is lost, even if they have not experienced trauma. But for a person who has experienced trauma, this can be critical to their experience of care.

Using knowledge of trauma to inform interactions

Being trauma informed should change how services are delivered and how patients are thought about and talked about. But it also requires us, as individual nurses and midwives, to be sensitive to the possibility of trauma in the lives of all patients we provide care to, and proactive in efforts to build safety and trust. This occurs in various ways and always needs to be adapted to the person. Considering the principles of TIC and how to enhance each in interactions may be helpful. It can also include how we introduce people to spaces and care, and how we move through those spaces with them. Many hospital and clinical spaces are not ideal, but offering choice where possible or considering the way spaces feel is important. When seeing patients in a hospital setting, I would start interactions by asking people where they would like to sit in the space and letting them know where most people choose to sit in case this helped them orient. Only once did a patient choose my desk chair over the other more usual choices and I went with it as it must have served some important purpose of power for them. This is a small moment in time, but it gives people choice, and it reduces shame. Offering this kind of choice is not always possible, but it is always possible to look around and identify what a person's experience might be. You don't need to know people's trauma history to anticipate and prevent challenges. For example, it is not necessary to know whether someone has been imprisoned to recognise the importance of people generally being able to see a doorway or window in most spaces. You don't need to know whether a person has been physically attacked to generally offer people an opportunity to sit somewhere with a wall behind them. Trauma informed interactions are about more than just us and our way of being; they are also about these practical things which can be crucial for people feeling safe enough to even begin to engage in care.

It is often in our first moments with a patient that we may sense what their internal state is. Are they seemingly shut down and hypo-aroused? Are they twitchy and hyper-aroused? Are they switching between these states? It is for us as nurses or midwives to support them to a regulated state. We do this through our therapeutic presence and by managing our own internal state.

The hospital waiting room where I worked was a highly dysregulating space for patients. Waiting rooms are pretty generic in hospitals, but many people are triggered by 'waiting'. It reenacts power dynamics and fear. It can remind people of waiting for help, waiting to be abused, or waiting for things to pass. People become agitated; they often can't wait or won't wait. They may fear being forgotten or ignored or feel strange and observed. Ideally, we set up better appointment systems, friendly waiting spaces, and more opportunity for power and control. But if we can't change these things, we can give people information and guidance on how long they will be waiting for and how they will know when it's their turn. One of the most trauma informed interactions I had with patients in that setting was sticking my head out of the office door and greeting them, smiling, and letting them know how long they may need to wait (Box 9.2).

Box 9.2: Vivienne and trauma in the waiting room

Vivienne is pregnant and attending the local public hospital for antenatal care. She generally avoids hospitals and healthcare because she doesn't like being in vulnerable situations. She would prefer not to receive any care but is worried that this may get her in trouble with child protection services. Vivienne grew up in an unpredictable household where there was violence and drug use. She used to lie awake as a child waiting to hear if her dad would come home drunk, and she would fear his violence if he did. She hasn't told the midwives this as she didn't think it was relevant to her pregnancy and because she fears judgement and assumptions that she might be a 'bad parent' by association. Vivienne is a single parent who is determined to try to give her baby a better childhood than she had, but she frequently feels judged by other parents for not having a partner. In the waiting area of the maternity unit, she is uncomfortable. There is an expectation that people will wait for appointments, and she observes couples sitting together. She feels like everyone else is a perfect family and this triggers shame. The act of waiting triggers her childhood fear, although she isn't consciously aware of this. She is agitated, pacing around the waiting area, and gets angry at the administrative staff. The midwives are busy and do not have time to deal with her behaviour, which they find difficult. The junior staff are scared of Vivienne and decide to wait until their senior colleague returns from lunch for Vivienne to be seen. What is happening to Vivienne is having a paradoxical effect. Her worries about being different and stared at are escalating, while her agitation is drawing attention to her. Waiting triggers her fear response, and this is leading to her having to wait longer. Her attempts to attend the hospital to avoid coming to the attention of authorities are leading to her being flagged as a potentially worrying parent.

One of the midwives approaches Vivienne and introduces herself and apologises for the extended wait. She explains to Vivienne that she will be seen by the senior midwife in half an hour. She offers Vivienne a quieter room to sit in if she would prefer and checks if she needs anything while she waits. She talks with Vivienne in a usual and friendly way. She notices that Vivienne has a book with her and says in an ordinary and friendly tone: 'your baby is so lucky to have a mum who likes to read'. She apologises that she has to return to her patients but asks Vivienne to let the midwife know at her appointment if there is anything that they could try with scheduling of future appointments so the staff could better support her. Without needing to know what Vivienne is experiencing or has experienced, the midwife responds to her in ways that recognised dysregulation, and promoted safety and trust. In introducing herself, noticing Vivienne's distress, offering options, observing strengths, and making plans for the future, she signals trustworthiness and a willingness to try to create safety.

Applying interpersonal neurobiology in practice

Interactions require connection. When the connection is effective, a co-regulation (and sometimes a co-dysregulation) occurs. There are a number of terms used to refer to the ways that our brains and bodies sync with other people's brains and bodies to reach such states of connection: 'attunement', 'synchrony', 'intersubjectivity', 'empathic resonance', 'neuro-reciprocity' (Isobel & Angus-Leppan, 2018), and so on. The idea is that our brains mimic the experiences of others when we tune into, or empathise with, their emotional state. On a brain level, the anterior insula, anterior cingulate cortex, and inferior frontal cortex, which activate when people experience an emotion, also activate when we see someone else experience an emotion. This process is thought to be mediated via the mirror neuron system. Similarly, on a body level, our breathing rates and heart rates can sync to other people who we are connected to, much in the same way that we might yawn if we see someone yawn. This happens in a variety of relationships.

The primary place where neuro-reciprocity first occurs is usually in parent-infant relationships. Infants are reliant upon caregivers to help them regulate their emotions, which requires caregivers to be able to attune to the infants' needs. The feeling of safety and trust fostered for infants through co-regulation of physiological states is the foundation for effective self-regulation. Such attunement also occurs in adult relationships, in intimate relationships, in friendships, in therapeutic relationships, and even in brief interactions. Neuro-reciprocity is not always about deep connection; it is also important for effective communication, collaboration, or shared tasks. For example, if I need to help you shuffle up your hospital bed, for the process to go smoothly, I attune to you. Perhaps I find myself holding my breath if you do, clenching my muscles, I absorb your worries and pain for a few minutes, and I notice shifts in your thoughts and affect. Then once you are settled, I return to my own homeostasis. But this interaction is bidirectional – if I am agitated and distracted as I shuffle you up the bed, you will likely feel more pain, you may feel more stressed, you attune to my state, and together we are dysregulated. If I am consciously slowing my breathing to a steady rate, relaxing my body, you will also feel more relaxed and calmer.

Therapeutic relationships can be part of physiological soothing for people who have experienced trauma. When people have experienced harm in relationships or have been in sustained states of hyper- or hypo-arousal, safe and buffering relationships which support them are incredibly powerful. While the interpersonal neurobiology of how we attune to others can sound complicated, actually we all know what it feels like to feel safe or unsafe in connection to others. It is felt almost immediately, although initial assumptions can subsequently be repaired or degraded. We can walk into a shop and feel safe, or feel judged. We can meet a health professional and immediately sense if they are overworked and grumpy. It's a felt sense that requires relational mindfulness, or being present in the interpersonal moment (Parnas & Isobel, 2019). Perhaps the most important trauma informed action we can take as nurses and midwives is to slow down, smile, hold a friendly soft face and gentle tone of voice, being ordinary and yet actively attending to safety in the interpersonal space.

The importance of co-regulation

In the same way that dysregulation of the nervous system in response to trauma makes sense, so does the importance of regulation. In the moments when we are dysregulated, it can be very difficult to think about what we need to return to a state of regulation. This is because it requires our pre-frontal cortex to be activated, and during survival responses the pre-frontal cortex is not activated. So, either we need to plan ahead for regulation strategies, or we may rely on habit or seek regulation from external people or things. We all have strategies we use to try to regulate ourselves, whether they are considered healthy or not. But when we can't access these, we rely on other humans to help us regulate through co-regulation.

The ways that we innately soothe babies are helpful to understand how co-regulation works to soothe distress. We may sway, or use rhythmic patting, rocking, repetitive low sounds, and so on, to soothe a distressed baby and soothe their nervous system dysregulation. When children are distressed and their needs are met, but they are seemingly out of control in their distress, we may hold them close to our bodies, wrap our arms around them, and repeat some sort of statement ('You are ok'), and we might remind them to breathe. As adults, we may not be as easily held and rocked, but our nervous systems still respond to similar stimuli. We might listen to music, or lie down and shut our eyes, or we might tap or wring our hands, or we might rock. It is not our role as nurses and midwives to hold and rock our patients, but the application of co-regulation to practice is awareness of our tone of voice, our breathing rate, our movements, and the 'energy' we bring into interactions. If we can keep our nervous systems regulated, our patients will be more regulated through interpersonal neurobiology. To be with someone who is distressed and to remain attuned to them but calm is one of the most soothing roles there is.

Polyvagal theory is one way to understand nervous system regulation

Polyvagal theory, developed by Dr. Stephen Porges (Porges, 2022), explains how our autonomic nervous system (ANS) influences our emotions and behaviours. The ANS controls many of our involuntary bodily functions like heart rate, digestion, and breathing through the sympathetic and parasympathetic systems. A key part of the theory is the Vagus nerve. The Vagus nerve is a part of the parasympathetic nervous system, extending from the brainstem to various organs, including the heart, lungs, and digestive tract. The 'theory' component relates to the links Porges has made between these systems and how they influence emotions and behaviours. According to Porges, when we feel safe, our ventral vagal pathway is active and we are calm, connected, and able to engage socially. When we perceive danger, our sympathetic system kicks in, preparing us to either fight or flight, and if the threat feels overwhelming, our vagal nerve pathway may cause us to freeze or shut down as a protective mechanism. In polyvagal theory, these responses are proposed to be hierarchical. This means that we work our way through them and move on to the next level when a strategy is ineffective.

Another relevant aspect of Porges' theory is the idea of neuroception. Neuroception is a neural process which is capable of distinguishing seen and felt cues of safety, danger, and threat. Through neuroception, Porges suggests that our nervous systems are constantly scanning the environment, beneath awareness, for possible sources of safety or threat. Sometimes we are aware of what the stimuli are that trigger neuroception responses (for example, a smile or a sudden movement), but other times we are only aware of our body's reactions, for example, a sudden feeling of unease or a feeling of social connectedness. This occurs without conscious awareness and influences how we respond to our environment and to people. Sources of threat or safety can be environmental but also interpersonal, for example, facial expressions. A friendly face and a smile are our most primal cues of safety, but there are many more in how we stand, speak, and look at patients.

Supporting trauma sensitivity via telehealth

The widespread uptake of telehealth has increased accessibility of services for people who may find it difficult or not possible to attend appointments. There can be concerns that safety can be harder to establish via telehealth. However, many people who have experienced trauma find telehealth safe-enough due to an enhanced sense of control. People can be less focused on their bodies and whether they are doing the right thing. There is also less interaction with other parts of care which can be triggering, like trying to find parking, running late, or waiting in areas.

It is obviously only in some areas of nursing and midwifery where telehealth is a possibility. In these settings, extra steps can support safety when there are reduced interpersonal visual cues. You may need to directly acknowledge the limitations of the space (e.g. 'I know it can be tricky on the phone, but I'm hoping we can talk a bit about...'), as well as describing your space so they can picture where you are (e.g. 'I'm calling you from my office at the hospital, there is no one else in the room') and also identify what may be difficult in this context (e.g. 'sometimes it can be hard for me to figure out what is happening for you when I can't see you, so if you need to take a break, please interrupt me to let me know'). Cues of safety and processes of empathy driven by mirror neurons still function across the video screens or phones, but the cues we get and give may be less clear. You may have to ask more directly, for example, 'I am wondering what you are feeling?' or 'I notice you seem distracted, is something happening for you right now?' and also narrate your own activities. For example, if you need to type while the person talks, let them know what you are doing and why. To facilitate attunement, if you are using video conferencing, it can be helpful to adjust your settings to just see the patient, close other pop-ups on your computer, and try to minimise multitasking, as while we may think we are still paying attention, distraction can be felt as rejection.

The final consideration relates to doing telehealth or video conferencing from home. During the Covid-19 pandemic, many healthcare workers who could work from home did. This meant sitting in their lounge rooms or kitchens and seeing patients virtually. I met many healthcare workers during this time who were experiencing work-related distress. If you spend the day at your kitchen table seeing patients, then at dinner time, they all sit metaphorically at the table with you. It is important to create some separation, both physically, where possible, by sitting in a certain spot in the house and psychologically by having end of the day and start of the day rituals to signal end points for our brains. This may be as small as shutting your laptop, packing it away, stretching, and saying goodbye to the space; anything to signal an end.

When trauma sensitive interactions don't have the desired effect

It is important not to assume that all trauma survivors are sensitive and misunderstood, and with a bit of kindness and therapeutic presence, they will open up, feel safe, and be grateful for our efforts. To be trauma sensitive is easy when it goes smoothly and is well-received, but to be informed about trauma is also to understand that it is not uncommon for people who have experienced trauma to be defensive, prickly, closed off, or hostile. These may all be trauma-related ways of interacting with the world and they make sense in the context of understanding trauma. So, while we can be trauma informed and sensitive with people who are distressed and want to be better understood, we also need to be trauma informed and sensitive with people who require healthcare but whose expressions of distress we may find uncomfortable or rejecting, or who do not want to be understood by us. In fact, these are the times that it is most important to be trauma informed and to try to stay present and non-reactive, asking ourselves, 'I wonder why this person may be responding in this way and is there anything I can do to try to make them feel more safe at this moment'. And then even if you don't know why, and even if you can't think of any way to make them feel safer, you have at least kept a lens of curiosity and empathy which will alter how you approach and interact with them.

Some people may feel very uncomfortable with close attention or questions about what they need. They may prefer us to just do the things we need to do and then leave them. Not everyone wants to be seen or noticed or cared for, and for some, asking what they need to feel safe or understood can feel unbearable. This requires us to notice and adapt our engagement accordingly. Being trauma informed can, at times, require us to be less attentive rather than more.

As professionals, the onus is on us to stay calm and polite, even under difficult circumstances. That doesn't mean we tolerate rudeness or verbal abuse, but it does mean that when patients are stressed or overwhelmed, we stay calm and curious and put in effort to connect.

Being sensitive to shame

Shame is often a persistent emotional state associated with trauma. Nathanson (1997) identified four responses to shame referred to as 'the compass of shame'. The four responses are interpersonal avoidance (denial, distraction, or substance use) or withdrawal (to stop people seeing our shameful selves or having the opportunity to judge or perceive us), defending against shame by attacking the self (with self-deprecation, self-blame, hatred, or actual harm) or by attacking others (distracting with blaming others, intimidation or twisting stories). Shame stops people from talking about trauma and stops people from engaging with services where trauma may be identified.

Some shame is inevitable. We can't always avoid accidentally activating people's shame within healthcare. However, it is our responsibility as healthcare workers to acknowledge shame, recognise it, and minimise its impacts. Shame is an activation of trauma, a defence against trauma, an effect of trauma, and a process by which healthcare may replicate trauma. Dolezal and Gibson (2022) identify a number of skills related to being sensitive to shame that they categorise as acknowledging, avoiding, and addressing.

Acknowledging shame

To acknowledge shame, we need to understand it. This includes why shame occurs, how it is evoked, why people hide shame, the embedded nature of shame in the self, and the complex ways that people have developed and refined to cope with shame. This also includes sensitivity to the ways that shame can be very well hidden, and that shaming can occur despite best intentions. Thus, as nurses and midwives, we need to be aware of subtle cues that might be clues that someone is experiencing shame. Some of these are well known, like blushing or looking away or guarding, and others are less recognisable, such as agitation or aggression or distracting. We also need to be careful to not let our own experiences of shame permeate interactions (Box 9.3).

Box 9.3: Clinical example of unintentional shaming

Consider a nurse who is changing a patient's soiled bedclothes on a general medical ward. The patient is making jokes and talking a lot, so the nurse assumes they are feeling comfortable. The patient says, 'I'm sure you see a lot of disgusting things in your job', while smiling. To make conversation and match the patient's demeanour, the nurse laughs and agrees.

This interaction could be unintentionally shaming. The patient is distracting from their own shame about the bedclothes while implying that they think it is disgusting, and the nurse, distracted by the incongruent affect, has agreed with the patient's worry that they are disgusting.

Perhaps the patient fell quiet after the nurse agreed and sat quietly looking out the window. Or perhaps their shoulders just dropped a little and they stopped smiling. If the nurse noticed this, they could repair this moment by saying something indirect like 'I don't find this disgusting at all' or even something direct like 'I don't want you to think that I find this sort of thing disgusting because I don't at all'.

Often, it isn't until after that we notice these small missteps. To be shame sensitive is to try to notice when people are giving subtle signs of possible shame. However, sometimes these only occur after shame has been activated.

Sometimes I think of shame as a funny little character. The character carries around a suitcase of jokes and tricks and distractions. It wears an oversized suit and is a skilled trickster, working hard to hide scars of trauma and to distract everyone from seeing the real them. It works so hard because it feels sure that the real them is inadequate, or flawed, or disgusting, or to blame. When I think of it this way, any aggression or distraction is viewed with empathy. Empathy for the part of the self that feels that way and that must work so hard to try to protect itself. Shame sensitive interactions are designed to not fall into the trick, to not get caught up in the act, but also not to dismantle the system or point out the strategy (thereby creating more shame). They are just ways of accepting, reassuring, and noticing.

Avoiding shaming

To avoid shame in interactions is to be conscious of the potential for shaming to occur, particularly where there are power differentials and vulnerability. Any patient in a healthcare context is expected to expose themselves to nurses and midwives. This occurs physically through undressing, lack of privacy, scrutinizing bodies and excretions, and psychologically through answering questions about their bodies, histories, and behaviours. Patients know that all these intimacies are scrutinised by healthcare providers and used to assess illness, recovery, and treatment efficacy. To avoid shame as much as possible in these interactions, we can pay attention to tone of voice, eye contact, body language, facial expressions, and words used. As nurses and midwives, we also need to be reflective about what assumptions we may hold and ways we may shame people through implications or judgements (Box 9.4).

Box 9.4: Clinical example of avoiding shame

A nurse needs to weigh a patient as part of an assessment. If the patient has a larger body, the nurse may quickly scan the patient with their eyes and then say, 'I'll just have to go grab the bigger scales'. The nurse may not be intending to shame the patient for their body size and instead has been just thinking logistically. Yet their dismissive tone, their body language, and their choice of words are inherently shaming. A few extra moments spent considering how interactions that require people's bodies, lives, or understanding to be scrutinised can be framed in ways that promote trust and safety is crucial. The nurse could have said nothing and just got the scales or could have said something less loaded like 'I will just go and grab a few things that I need'. They could also have minimised attention on the person's size at all, saying something like 'we have to weigh everyone who comes to this clinic, is that ok with you?' I also note here that it shouldn't only be people in larger bodies who get this approach as that is also stigmatising. Many people struggle with shame about their bodies being too small, too big, too long, too short, too lumpy, too smelly, or too weird. As nurses and midwives, we have an obligation to avoid shaming in relation to bodies at all.

Avoiding shaming also extends to how we talk about our patients, how we accept other people talking about our patients, how we represent the work that we do, and how we understand the role of context in people's experiences of health and illness. This might mean not joining in on jokes, sharing examples of our work with care, and pushing back on discourses that shame individuals or groups.

Addressing shame

Addressing shame requires us to help people identify shame and work through it. This needs to always be a trauma informed process that prioritises safety. Patients often confide in nurses and midwives about things they feel shame about, giving us an opportunity to help them address them. Being able to hear people's experiences and gently question the shame attached to them can allow people to feel unburdened. It is a process of shining a light on things that look scarier in the dark (Box 9.5).

Box 9.5: Clinical example of addressing shame

Imagine that a patient with gestational diabetes tells her midwife that she has not been following the diet that has been suggested. She might cautiously say 'I haven't been that good this week with what I've eaten'. Rather than buying into the dichotomy of 'good' and 'bad', the midwife may recognise through the patient's stammering and their offering of an aligned emotion (embarrassment) that the patient is feeling shame about this. The midwife could immediately respond with warmth and curiosity by saying something like 'It sounds like you have had a hard week' or 'Tell me about the week'. They could also challenge the self-shaming directly by saying something like 'Lots of people find this diet so challenging. Which bits did you manage to maintain this week?' It is important to note here that directly calling out shame can be quite shaming in itself. This means avoiding saying assumptive or offering any reassurance directly such as 'you don't need to feel shame'. Shame is designed to disguise itself, and pointing out its disguise can be too confronting.

Sometimes patients tell us directly about their shame. For example, they may say 'I'm so ashamed that you have to help me with this' or 'I hate that you are seeing me like this'. In these moments, people are giving us an opportunity to respond in ways that address shame. Not through reassurance or dismissal but by challenging the idea that these are things to be ashamed of at all. For example, we can say 'It is a privilege to be able to help you like this/see you like this' or 'In my role I get to see people who need help in lots of different ways or are vulnerable in lots of different ways, this is some of what makes my job so incredible'. At other times, people may drop hints about shame, and we may need to pick up the clues and help them make sense of their experiences (Box 9.6).

Box 9.6: Clinical example of addressing shame

I saw a woman who felt terrible about how she had acted in the days leading up to the birth of her baby. She was teary on the postnatal ward and kept apologising to her partner for what she described as 'acting so crazy'. She had taken to her bed in the days leading up to the birth and had not been interacting. At one stage, she said she didn't care if the baby came or not. Despite her partner's reassurance and her obvious connection to the baby now, she was obviously distressed, and I wondered if she felt shame for the things she had said. In addressing this shame directly, I said something like: 'sometimes people tell terrible stories to themselves about what it means that they said something awful when they were in pain or scared. In my role, I see so many people who are in pain or scared and I can assure you, many people say things they don't mean or things that they think they "mean at that moment but later don't think anymore"'. I could see her eyes meet mine, and I glimpsed the shame in her face. We had a chance together to talk about the shame, to shine the torch on all the worst thoughts she was having, and address the shame head-on (Box 9.7).

Box 9.7: Clinical example of addressing shame

Another pregnant woman I saw had intrusive thoughts of her baby being injured. The thoughts were stemming from anxiety and were distressing in themselves. But there was something else going on. She found it hard to talk about her thoughts even though she desperately wanted help. In my office, I watched her fight a battle with herself. She covered her eyes, she scratched at her fingernails, she sighed deeply, she couldn't look at me, and she spoke so quietly I had to lean in to hear. She was feeling terrible shame about these thoughts. So, then she had two problems screaming at her: the thoughts and the shame about the thoughts. Intrusive thoughts are a real poster child of shame. They present you with your worst nightmare or the most embarrassing or shocking thing you can imagine, and they keep shoving it in front of your mind in a way that can feel overwhelming. But the less you talk about the thoughts and the more you try to push them away and bury them under shame – the more power they get. In this context, shame is like a street performer who won't let you walk past until you watch the show and give them some money. In holding the shame with care and talking to my patient about how intrusive thoughts are the things you are most scared of, and no, they didn't make me think she was a bad mother; in fact, they gave me a little insight into how much she wanted to keep her baby safe in the world; they slowly lost their power.

Shame is inherent to so much of what is pervasive and difficult about trauma. Shame is part of what embeds trauma into the self and changes how people perceive themselves in relation to others. Of course, there is also fear and betrayal and hypervigilance and mistrust. But shame is also a decoy for all of these things. And like many of these concepts, they are not discrete but overlap. Shame is one of the most prominent and tangible outcomes of trauma. It is also something we all understand the feeling of, regardless of trauma. We can recall a time when we have felt shame- shame about our behaviour, shame about our body, shame about a reaction we had, or not understanding something, shame about not knowing how to fit in or act, and shame about wanting something we can't have or not wanting something we do have. We can take this understanding of how shame feels to try to minimise shame in our practice.

Reflective functioning and understanding the inner world of others

This seems like a helpful spot to mention the concept of 'reflective functioning'. Reflective functioning refers to our capacity to understand the mental state of others. It's a complex process that allows us to think about ourselves and other people as psychological beings who are driven by their own underlying motivations, thoughts, beliefs, and feelings. It is essentially a curiosity or wondering about the inner world of other people. We may ask ourselves: 'I wonder why they responded in that way, maybe they felt....' Or similarly, we may reflect on ourselves and think: 'I think I reacted that way because I felt....' To be curious about the cognitive processes of other people is not about mind reading or assuming, but instead about paying attention and attempting to understand. It is also linked to our ability to cope with difficult events. For example, your co-worker may be rude to you, and while you are offended, you may think, 'I know they've been really stressed lately and we usually get along well, so perhaps they reacted that way because of things going on in their life'.

Reflective functioning is the process that underlies this 'making a guess' about what is happening for someone. It requires empathy and regulation skills and is a skill developed throughout childhood and refined throughout adulthood. It starts to develop in infancy when our caregivers reflect our emotions back to us, soothe us, and help us cope with them. For example, a caregiver may say to a crying baby, 'Oh you are so sad', and then offer reassurance and soothing, and we learn through repeated interactions that what we feel is sadness and that it is manageable. Then, as children, perhaps we see someone who is crying and we know that they are sad and that they will be ok. Maybe our caregiver gets sad, and it makes us sad, but they tell us it's ok they are sad because of something to do with work and not anything that we did, and then we give them a pat to model soothing. We are learning that people have their own unique emotions, for reasons, and this affects their behaviour, but it isn't all to do with us. Imaginative play is also important for this process, as children often play games where they make their toys or adults cry or angry or have a surprise party, or they pretend to scare us, as ways of playing with and understanding how people experience and express emotion.

This is relevant to TIC in a few ways. The first is that to be trauma informed requires us to have and use reflective functioning to try to understand why people may be responding the way that they are. The next is that trauma can interfere with the development of reflective functioning. If people grow up in contexts where they don't have people reflecting back their emotions, helping them make sense of them and manage them, and opportunities to play, they may not develop this skill. Disruption to attachment relationships prior to about the age of 5 can interrupt the development of reflective functioning. But trauma after this age also can, if it becomes not safe to try to understand people around us, or understanding the motivations of people who hurt us feels incomprehensible. A trauma adaptation can be to not develop reflective functioning, or a trauma impact can be to not have the opportunities to.

There are usually clues in the ways that people speak that can let us know that they may lack reflective functioning; for example, they may be defensive when asked about why things have occurred ('how should I know??') or they may give overly simple summaries of situations ('our marriage is perfect, there are never any issues at all') or they may deflect answers about other people's motives ('you better ask them that'). Of course, we all do these things sometimes. But we all usually also take guesses at things which indicates reflective functioning capability, for example, 'I'm not sure why that patient did that? Maybe they thought I wasn't going to notice' or 'I just got so annoyed at that patient, I must need a lunch break'. In these examples, whether the reason is 'right' or not is not important; the key thing is that we are trying to link an emotion or behaviour to an underlying motivation. This is reflective functioning. The good news is that reflective functioning is something we can all improve on throughout life, so it isn't fixed.

The final reason I mention reflective functioning here is that when we need reflective functioning the most, it is least accessible to us. Our stress response can override our capacity to think about other people. We all experience this, for example, we are having a bad day and we feel hard done by and we start to see the worst in other people's behaviour towards us. We gather evidence to add to the way that we already feel. Or perhaps someone cuts us off in traffic and we feel rage. We don't usually stop to wonder what makes them in a hurry and whether there may be reasons that they need to get in front of us.

This is part of why we need to become aware of our own reactivity in the healthcare context. We need to notice when we are stressed and overwhelmed and it is making it hard to be present. We need to take a moment to regroup ourselves and we need to see our roles as nurses and midwives to use our reflective functioning to enable us to be present and engaged with our patients, despite what might have happened to them in their lives.

Relational ruptures and disconnects

In any interaction or relationship, there will be moments of disconnect or 'rupture' of attunement. Being trauma informed does not require you to be perfect, but rather to notice ruptures or disconnects and make efforts to repair.

Ruptures or disconnects can be momentary or more significant. They can happen for many reasons. Two examples that I have observed across healthcare repeatedly are when people interact with services in ways that we find difficult and they may get labelled as 'manipulative' or some other word with negative connotations. This happens quite a lot in mental health settings, but I have seen it in other contexts too. It usually happens when people seek to get their needs met by services in ways that do not fit the expected pathway; for example, they may ask multiple nurses for something in different ways, and we might say, 'I already told her she couldn't leave the ward to go to the shop this morning, so why is she asking you again?' This example has some nuance ... perhaps the afternoon staff always have a more flexible approach, or perhaps it is always busy in the morning on the ward, so the afternoon is a better time to ask. Or maybe the person really needed a tampon or personal item but didn't want to ask the staff for that. Or perhaps the person saw their doctor in between those two requests and the doctor had altered their leave status, or maybe it is not clear on the unit how often you can ask about going to the shop. Regardless, people often have learnt and use complex strategies to get their needs met. We all manipulate sometimes, and in positions of powerlessness, this may be amplified.

There is trauma knowledge that also underpins this. In untraumatised childhoods, children have their needs met without needing to work to do so. Adults bring food, shelter, love, delight, and safety as part of their expected roles. In situations of trauma, abuse, or neglect, children need to develop new ways to survive and to get these basic needs met. People are incredibly good at finding ways to survive their circumstances. Over a lifetime, this can mean that they function in ways that seem out of the norm but are normal to them. For example, if you grew up with parents who took drugs and sometimes responded positively and sometimes negatively to you, you would learn to choose who you asked what, when. If you grew up in a situation where you only received care and affection when you were highly distressed, you would learn to know when to express distress to ensure you received care. Through a trauma informed lens, if people have to 'manipulate' us to get their needs met, it is important to be compassionate to why they may have had to develop in such a way that this is how they have learnt that they will get their needs met. But we also need to make sure the 'problem' isn't us or the system.

This is also associated with the idea of 'splitting'. Splitting occurs (theoretically) when patients, either unconsciously or consciously, create divisions within the treating team. It can occur because the patient identifies one staff member as 'good' and others as 'bad', so always asks the 'good' one for assistance and doesn't engage with the others. In psychological terms, splitting is usually seen as a reflection of the patient's internal state and learnt defence mechanisms. It can be framed as a way of having control or protecting the self through alliances. It can also be framed as projecting their own internal struggles for power and control onto the team. Splitting as a phenomenon is surely based on some truth, but the reality of many healthcare settings is that often the issue is not the patient. Our teams are frequently inconsistent; we can all identify who are the 'nicer' nurses or doctors on our teams and it makes sense to imagine that we would all learn to ask the people who are more likely to say yes. As nurses and midwives, we are all likely also aware that there are often staff politics playing out in teams. When splitting occurs, it usually occurs down already established cracks in teams or in places where there are tensions, a lack of communication or teamwork occurring, or existing misuses of power or lack of transparency. Reflecting on what challenges exist within our teams and noticing how these are highlighted through the ways patients learn to interact with us should be the first step, long before we ever decide that someone is 'manipulative'. A critical part of being trauma informed is recognising all the ways that people who experience trauma get blamed for things that are not, and were never, their fault. As professionals, it is important that we take responsibility for the impact we have on people in our interactions. At a minimum, this requires us to meaningfully apologise for the distress we cause (Box 9.8).

Box 9.8: Clinical examples of repairing a relational rupture by apologising in the moment

Grace is an inpatient on a postnatal ward in a large hospital. Her midwife for the morning is Ana. Ana has built a good rapport with Grace and has noticed Grace starting to relax in her company. Grace has an Apprehended Violence Order out against her ex-partner and father of her new baby due to violence. Her ex-partner is not allowed on the ward. Mostly Ana has avoided talking about this situation as the Social Worker is involved and Ana has been more focussed on supporting Grace with baby care. As Ana is swaddling the baby and they are chatting, Ana is facing away from Grace leaning over the bassinet. She is explaining to Grace the technique for swaddling as Grace laughs about how last night she had tried to do it and the baby came unwrapped immediately. Ana says 'Oh my goodness my husband used to be the absolute worst; he couldn't wrap our baby at all. I was almost better off without him'.

Ana freezes. She had been trying to share something from her own life to aid the connection, but straight after she says it, she realises it may have been insensitive. She notices Grace has gone quiet. Ana keeps fussing over the baby. Her face feels red, and she is distracted by her own internal critical monologue ('why did you say THAT?'; 'why do you always say thoughtless things?'; 'You have to get out of here'). She turns back to Grace, handing her the baby. She can see that Grace is shut down, her eyes are looking downward, and even though she smiles a bit at Ana, she looks like she might cry. Ana realises she needs to repair this rupture. She softens her face and sits next to Grace, and turning to look her in the eyes, she says, 'I'm sorry I said that about my husband Grace. I wasn't thinking. I can only imagine how hard it must be for you at the moment'. Then she sits quietly. She notices Grace soften in her posture and turn to look at Ana; she has tears in her eyes, but the connection is tentatively repaired (Boxes 9.9 and 9.10).

Box 9.9: Clinical example of repairing a disconnect without addressing it directly

Ana is helping Katie to have a shower. Katie had a baby 3 days ago via caesarean section and is requiring support to shower. Ana has been caring for Katie every day, and they have been getting along well. Ana likes Katie; they are similar types of people and interacting feels easy. Today in the bathroom, Katie asks Ana to face the other way while she showers. Ana is offended by this rejection of her clinical presence. She doesn't say anything, but her face and body posture stiffen. She turns away and thinks about how this is her job, and she sees vulnerable bodies every day. She feels rejected by Katie. She crosses her arms and sighs. When Katie indicates she is comfortable for Ana to turn around, Ana turns with a stern face and her voice is hurried. She sees Katie flinch and pull her towel tighter around herself as though protecting her body from Ana. Ana pauses and refocuses on the interaction. She uncrosses her arms, slows her breathing, and smiles. She makes sure her voice is friendly in tone. She says, 'Sometimes people feel like strangers in their own bodies after having a baby. How did it feel to shower?' She looks at Katie's face and makes sure to soften her expression and gaze. She feels Katie's posture soften. Katie breathes out and starts to talk about how she feels about her body after birth.

Box 9.10: Clinical example of repairing a disconnect after it has resolved

Ana has a student nurse called Violet with her for the rest of her shift. Violet is nervous and requires a lot of reassurance and support. Violet is a similar age to Ana's own daughter. Ana remembers what it is like to be a student, so she usually has a lot of patience with students, but there is something about Violet that really irritates her. Violet seems distracted and doesn't really seem to listen when Ana talks to her. As the afternoon goes on, Ana finds herself avoiding Violet, leaving Violet to read notes rather than assist with tasks and speaking to her in a patronising and abrupt tone. Ana goes on her tea break, and when she returns, she can't locate Violet. Later, the midwifery unit manager says to Ana, 'Ana, your student was really having a hard time, so I have reallocated her to someone else for the rest of the shift. Let's catch up about it tomorrow.' Ana is fuming. She can't believe that Violet has now got her in trouble with management. All evening, she is feeling angry and finds herself complaining about Violet and the injustice of it with her family. Over dinner, her daughter says, 'I feel for Violet, I have to deal with that every day!' Ana rolls her eyes but this comment stays in her mind. The next morning, when she meets with the manager and Violet, she apologises for having been short with Violet the day prior. She explains she had been tired and was finding the day a bit challenging. She says she remembers what it is like to be a student, and she apologises for making Violet feel like she was in the way. Violet has hunched shoulders and is looking at the floor, but she looks up a little and makes eye contact with Ana. Ana smiles and says, 'I am really sorry I made you feel that way'.

References

Dolezal, L., & Gibson, M. (2022). Beyond a trauma-informed approach and towards shame-sensitive practice. *Humanities and Social Sciences Communications*, 9(1), 214. https://doi.org/10.1057/s41599-022-01227-z

Isobel, S., & Angus-Leppan, G. (2018). Neuro-reciprocity and vicarious trauma in psychiatrists. *Australasian Psychiatry, 26*(4), 388–390. https://doi.org/10.1177/1039856218772223

Nathanson, D. L. (1997). *Affect theory and the compass of shame.* In M. R. Lansky & A. P. Morrison (Eds.), *The widening scope of shame* (pp. 107–138). Analytic Press.

Parnas, S., & Isobel, S. (2019). Using relational mindfulness to facilitate safety in the clinical encounter. *Australasian Psychiatry, 27*(6), 596–599. https://doi.org/10.1177/1039856219866318

Porges, S. W. (2022). Polyvagal theory: A science of safety. *Frontiers in Integrative Neuroscience, 16,* 871227. https://doi.org/10.3389/fnint.2022.871227

10 Trauma informed interventions

Being trauma informed in practice requires attention to what we do, but also how we go about doing it. Sometimes we can't alter the 'what we have to do' bit, but we can always alter the 'how we go about doing it' bit. This is where the informed part of being trauma informed comes in. If we understand what trauma is and we understand the diverse ways it can impact people and impact healthcare, then we need to think about how we can adapt our care to be sensitive to this.

In many parts of nursing and midwifery, we engage closely with people's bodies. We touch people to perform clinical tasks, and we are generally more intimate with other people's bodies than occurs in other social and professional contexts. As students, it can take time to feel comfortable touching, washing, looking at, and intervening with bodies, yet over time we often become somewhat 'desensitised'. As people around us may ask, 'how do you do your job?', we shrug and smile. Because part of nursing and midwifery is retaining the humanity and dignity of people, while becoming somewhat detached from the tasks we are undertaking. Historically, nursing has valued emotional detachment and professional distancing as ways of engaging with the body, separate from the person. In doing so, there is always a risk that we might forget how it is for our patients. For anyone, having their body observed, talked about, or touched in a medical setting can be uncomfortable, embarrassing, or shameful. However, for people who have experienced trauma, it can be triggering, overwhelming, or lead them to avoid medical care. While this occurs during intrusive care of parts of our bodies we consider 'private', it can also occur from any intervention.

When I was working in an antenatal setting, my office was opposite the clinic room where urine testing and other physical assessments such as weighing occurred. Pregnant women needed to come to the door of the clinic room and wait for a midwife to appear and then ask to have their urine tested or to be weighed, as part of their routine antenatal care. I knew the midwives who worked there well, and they were all kind and skilled. Yet I heard many interactions from my office that I knew would trigger shame. Women getting in trouble for putting their urine sample in the wrong spot, comments made about urine colours and whether women were drinking enough water, women unsure how to ask about the details of what they were meant to do with their urine collection device, women who didn't want to be weighed, women whose weight was commented on … and so on. I knew that there was no intended malice in these interactions; the midwives were in their 'work mode', where the bodies were vessels for carrying the babies, and their job was to screen and monitor. But within this was an intimacy, the things that come out of our bodies are intimate, the things we need to do and share about our bodies are intimate, and the process of presenting our bodies to be

DOI: 10.4324/9781003530770-13

examined is intimate. And within all of these interactions, which would occur prior to any appointment where bodies would actually be poked and prodded and measured and examined, there was a need for trauma sensitivity.

And of course, then there is all of the washing and looking and touching and talking about that we do. Touch in nursing can occur for different purposes. Touch occurs as part of a procedure or treatment, for example, holding someone's arm while administering an injection. Touch can be used to communicate empathy and care, for example, putting your hand on someone's shoulder or patting their foot as you leave. O'Lynn and Krautscheid (2011) define 'intimate touch' in a nursing context as touching areas of people's bodies for task-oriented purposes, particularly those areas which may lead to discomfort, anxiety, or fear, such as genitalia, buttocks, perineum, inner thighs, lower abdomen, and breasts. They asked members of the public what nurses could do to make them feel less worried about intimate touch and how to enhance feelings of respect and dignity. While they didn't focus on trauma survivors, this research provides important clues about how to be trauma informed. The researchers found that, excluding in emergencies, people want clear communication, choice, and dignity. People want to know before intimate touch is undertaken why it is necessary and what it involves. They expect nurses to seek permission before initiating touch, and they want to be involved in deciding when and how it occurs. These seem like basic approaches, but it is the conscious attention to ensuring they occur that is important and, for trauma survivors, essential. It makes sense that intimate touch would be challenging for people who have experienced sexual trauma, but the vulnerability, exposure, and power differential can make the experience a challenge for trauma survivors of any kind. To be trauma informed is to use this approach with anyone and any touch in the healthcare context, in case the person has experienced trauma but also because the approach can benefit anyone.

Preventing triggers during interventions

In any nursing or midwifery intervention, there is a risk of triggering trauma. It is impossible to avoid all sensory experiences that may trigger a flashback or other physical reaction. There is no quick way to remove triggers, and it is a significant misunderstanding of trauma to imagine that you can avoid triggering someone just by being careful. While some trauma triggers are clear (for example, intrusive procedures or talking about violence), many are much more subtle. Triggers may be a facial expression, a turn of phrase, a smell, or a feeling. Our role as nurses and midwives is to reduce exposure to likely triggers, recognise when people may be being triggered, support people to return to a place of safety anchored in the present if they are triggered, support people to identify what their triggers may be, and develop safety plans to minimise their impacts.

Some examples of ways we can prevent triggers are by paying attention to the clinical environment. Perhaps there are things that may obviously be triggering for people, such as a lack of privacy or unclear instructions. In our interactions, we can reduce the likelihood of triggering people by explaining procedures or expectations clearly, paying attention to our voice and body language, seeking consent before touching people, and paying attention to the person in front of us. Another very good way is to ask people, 'Is there anything we can do to make you more comfortable while you are here?' or 'Are there things that it is helpful for us to know in delivering care to you?'

People can't always articulate their triggers. They may not even know them. Part of being trauma informed is that we pay attention and notice shifts in people's level of arousal or engagement. We might notice a change in someone's behaviour or demeanour, if they seem to withdraw or become agitated or start breathing quickly or get an unfocused gaze. The most immediate task is not to point this out but to try to support the person to return to the present by adjusting our own presence to match the desired energy (for example, if they seem distant, you may start moving around more, whereas if they seem agitated, you might slow yourself down). You may pause what you are doing or try to support grounding through offering a drink of water or a break. You might check in with the patient and say, 'I just noticed you seemed to get more ... is everything ok?' or you might ask what they need from you. We need to pay attention to our tone of voice, our body language, and our facial expression. We may try to reorient to the present by narrating the immediate things happening ('I will just finish this form and then we can move to doing this other thing'). It may be helpful to revisit the conversation later, saying 'I noticed that last time or earlier you seemed to get ... when I did ... Do you think there is anything we could do to make it easier for you next time?' The focus should be on the care context and what the person needs from you or what resources within themselves they can access if the same thing were to occur again. We can help people identify things that help them in the moment as well, for example, acceptance that triggers may occur and that it is ok because the system that gets activated is the same one that has kept them safe in the past; we could try taking deep breaths, squeezing something, having someone with us, distracting ourselves, or doing whatever works in the moment and then making time later to reflect about what might have caused it.

Back when computer games were fairly new, I used to play a game called minesweeper. You had to click on squares and try to avoid clicking on the squares that hid a bomb. At first, it was luck; you just had to start clicking. But there was also logic that developed. When you clicked on squares that weren't mines, you got an indication of how many mines were nearby. Knowledge became your tool. You could just keep clicking wildly and hoping for the best, but by identifying the patterns and using the information, you could get through the game safely. Managing trauma triggers can feel like playing minesweeper – you carefully navigate uncertain ground, over time coming to better anticipate where potential triggers might be, but there are also always ones that surprise you. While minesweeper relies on logic and deduction, managing trauma triggers combines awareness, coping strategies, and experience. A crucial part is monitoring ourselves also, as it can be hard to stay present and engaged when someone else is triggered. It takes time to regulate ourselves so we can help regulate others.

It is also important to note that being trauma informed requires awareness that the ways trauma impacts people are not linear and predictable. I met a woman who was pregnant and had a history of child sexual abuse who did not find internal vaginal examinations or being asked about her history of abuse triggering, even if she didn't like these experiences. However, she did experience intense panic attacks associated with her baby's movements inside her. This example is a reminder that while information or content or things can be distressing or remind us of other things, what 'triggers' the unconscious activation of fear response systems is often unpredictable.

Even though trauma informed care isn't one set thing, in some ways when you start trying to write examples of what it looks like in practice, they all end up being the same. Foster safety, be kind and communicative, collaborate, ask permission, notice shifts in arousal, support regulation … these are the heart of what it is to be trauma informed while you undertake interventions of any kind. It is the intentionality that makes it different from usual care. Attention to the person and their state of regulation, attention to ourselves and cues of safety or dangers, using transparency, and attending to power.

Box 10.1: Clinical example of a midwifery intervention

Jean is 32 weeks pregnant with her second baby. Her first baby was born still at term. Jean presents to the delivery unit with reduced foetal movements and is assessed by the midwife on duty. Jean has presented a number of times and the staff are getting frustrated. However, protocol is that a detailed history and examination is undertaken. The midwife introduces herself to Jean and immediately offers reassurance that they will do an ultrasound and check on the baby. She reassures Jean that her concerns are important and that they will work together to assess the situation. The midwife listens attentively as Jean describes her concerns about reduced foetal movements and shows her the diary she has been keeping about movements. The midwife checks whether Jean is experiencing any other symptoms such as pain or bleeding. She says, 'I can see from your notes about the loss of your last baby. I'm so sorry'. She informs Jean that she has access to the notes and doesn't need any further information unless there is anything Jean wants to tell her. Jean says in a snappy tone that her baby's name was Sam.

Before getting the ultrasound machine, the midwife says, 'I can imagine this feels scary after what you've been through with Sam; is there any way I could support you more while we do the ultrasound?' Jean is a bit dismissive of the midwife and tells her she's been through it before and she just wants to 'get on with it'. She looks away. The midwife doesn't react; she just narrates what will happen next and the plan for monitoring. She pays close attention to Jean's face and body language. At one point, she carefully puts her hand on Jean's shoulder and sees how Jean reacts. Jean clings to her hand but doesn't say anything. The midwife continues with the monitoring without speaking until they locate the baby's heart rate and Jean's body relaxes.

Reflection on Box 10.1

- In many ways, this is an unremarkable interaction, much like any other that may occur. However, trauma sensitivity is woven through it in ways that may not be apparent.
- The midwife takes Jean's concerns seriously, and if she feels annoyed, she doesn't let that show. This takes self-regulation and is important for establishing safety.
- The midwife acknowledges the information she has access to and her awareness of the loss of Sam, while giving Jean a chance to share more if she wants. This fosters transparency and trust.
- The midwife draws links between what happened with Sam and how Jean may be feeling right now, with a focus on how the midwife can make her feel more comfortable and safe in the current care context.
- The midwife stays focused on the relational space, noticing how Jean looks and responds and trying to adapt her own behaviour and demeanour to match Jean's. This supports co-regulation.

Trauma informed invasive procedures

In nursing and midwifery practice, people often require interventions that are invasive. Invasive procedures can be anything that violate a person's bodily boundary, whether it's the use of a tongue depressor to check a sore throat or a scope of an intimate orifice. Nurses and midwives may undertake these procedures or assist others in undertaking them. Invasive procedures are a crucial time for trauma sensitive practice.

Box 10.2: Clinical example of an invasive procedure

Please read Hannah's story. Hannah is a survivor of child sexual abuse.

> I had to get my IUD removed and a new one inserted; I'd been putting it off because I was dreading it. I find the process so intrusive and upsetting. Even though I have had a lot of trauma therapy and I feel like I can mostly manage myself and my responses, it hasn't taken away the memories that my body and mind hold. Any procedure that involves taking off my clothes is difficult. I tried to think of ways to get out of it but I have medical reasons for needing the IUD, and even if I didn't, trauma has taken so much from me; I refuse to let it take medical care or contraception options from me too.

> The doctor seemed nice enough, sort of business like but warm. She didn't ask me anything about how I was feeling about the procedure or if I needed anything, so I didn't say anything about how nervous I was. She seemed a little bit in a rush, and I didn't want to be a nuisance. She told me to take off my underpants and lie on the table and covered me with a very small and thin disposable cloth. It didn't feel like it covered me at all. I started to feel nervous. She said she was going to get the nurse who would assist and she left the door a tiny bit ajar as she left. I felt very exposed. My naked bits were facing the door and through the crack at the side of the door I watched for any movement, any sign of someone walking from the waiting room to the toilet opposite this room. I felt like that cloth offered me no safety or dignity.

> The doctor and the nurse returned. I didn't hear the nurse's name if she said it as she had a mask on. When she entered the room, she started talking to the doctor about how she had slipped on the driveway of the surgery the night before and how the practice manager needed to arrange cleaning of the moss on the driveway to ensure no one else got hurt. She kept talking as if I wasn't there, detailing her grazes and bruises from her fall. I wondered if she was trying to make an awkward situation less awkward by signalling how unfazed she was by my nakedness. But her lack of attention to me and the situation felt strange.

> The doctor said 'I'm just going to check your uterus before we start' and suddenly inserted a finger in my vagina. I flinched and made a noise of surprise. I hadn't realised that was what she meant. 'Just relax' she told me. I covered my face with my hands and shut my eyes. The nurse was standing next to my head. Maybe she was noticing my distress and trying to distract me, or maybe she was just chatting inanely, I'm not sure, but either way she just kept talking:

complimenting my nail polish, talking about the weather, saying how well I was doing. I couldn't respond. The doctor seemed a bit annoyed by this 'Hannah, you don't need to cover your face. Hannah, we want you to talk to us so we know you are ok'. 'I'm ok', I managed to reply.

As she undertook the procedure, I kept my eyes shut and tried to focus on my breathing. I remember thinking to myself that I was doing ok … I was getting through it. I flinched numerous times and I heard the doctor say 'you are very sensitive'. This comment was jarring. Am I? Wouldn't anyone be?

The nurse was still next to my head offering constant reassuring statements about how well I was doing. I could feel how uncomfortable she was with my discomfort. Her dismissal and reassurance felt like a demand of me to do well. She offered me her hand to squeeze and I held it gratefully. She told me the doctor was just cleaning up the area as the procedure was mostly done and I wondered what she meant. Did I need cleaning? Was I dirty? Does everyone need cleaning?

And then, it was done. The nurse called me a good girl, told me I'd done really well, patted my head and walked out of the room, leaving the doctor to finalise the procedure and help me up. I felt glad it was over. I felt like, all things considered, I had done ok. I had felt alone and violated and in pain, but I had coped. Thinking about this now, I can see how this had replicated my abuse, even though both the doctor and nurse were kind and meant well. Tears rolled down my cheeks as I sat in the chair and the doctor completed the consult. The tears felt embarrassing. They were betraying how I thought I felt. The doctor noticed 'You are crying!' she seemed shocked. She handed me a tissue. Her eyes looked concerned. She asked if I was in pain and suggested I take more pain relief. I didn't say anything. I felt ashamed of my tears, ashamed of my 'sensitivity', ashamed of my body and ashamed of what had just happened. Now that the procedure was over, I just wanted to get out of there with no further conversation. I didn't want her to ask any questions or try to understand. And so that was that. I stepped out into the sun, made sure not to slip on the mossy driveway as I walked away, and I never went back for the scheduled follow-up.

In Box 10.2, Hannah describes in detail the interactions and how she experienced them. I can't help but wonder how the doctor or nurse would feel if they read this account – would they be annoyed? Would they be surprised? These accounts can be hard for us to hear as health professionals, as we can feel defensive. None of us goes to work to cause harm or trauma to people. We all would have different accounts of the events and likely want to explain all the things we did to try to put Hannah at ease. Perhaps we would go so far as to start to say how 'difficult' Hannah was as a patient. But part of becoming trauma informed requires openness to the ways that people can experience us, despite our good intentions.

It feels apparent that neither the doctor nor the nurse in Hannah's story was particularly trauma informed. That isn't to say they weren't kind or professional or that they didn't do things that provided comfort to Hannah, like offering a hand to hold or a tissue. The nurse stayed close to Hannah's head, tried to build rapport, used distraction, and noticed Hannah's distress. These are all aspects of good practice. Not being trauma informed doesn't always equate to bad practice; it can just mean limited awareness of how a person may be experiencing an intervention and missed opportunities to create safety.

If we consider how it could have been different if this procedure had been undertaken in a way informed by trauma, we need to remember that it isn't always appropriate to ask directly about trauma. Defensive practitioners often retort to the suggestion of a need to be trauma informed with statements about how they don't have time to ask about trauma or they don't want to distress people by asking about trauma. This is not what is required. I have no doubt that the doctor was allocated a short period of time to insert Hannah's IUD and opening up a conversation about childhood trauma would have been unwise. Hannah likely also would not have wanted to disclose her history of child sexual abuse at that moment as she was actively trying to work to manage her risk of retraumatisation and bringing up memories of the abuse would have been counterproductive.

But there were opportunities for the doctor and nurse to have enough understanding of trauma that they could signal attentiveness and safety for Hannah without asking directly about abuse. For example, by asking prior to commencing what Hannah needed to feel comfortable and by indicating how Hannah could communicate her needs throughout by seeking consent prior to touching or violating Hannah's bodily boundaries.

The intrusive nature of the procedure left Hannah vulnerable to shame. The comments about being sensitive or needing cleaning were likely well-intentioned but were highly likely to cause shame. Knowledge of trauma may have enabled the doctor and nurse to identify the possibility that Hannah may have experienced sexual violence in her life and to be actively shame-minimising in their approach. Their use of language could have carefully avoided any blaming, shaming, or patronising words. Hannah felt her coping mechanisms of covering her face and keeping quiet were bothering the doctor and nurse, who wanted her to uncover her face and answer their questions. A trauma informed lens would have allowed them to recognise these actions as techniques she had developed to cope with traumatic experiences. They could have agreed on alternate ways to identify 'if she was ok' rather than compromising the things she needed to do to cope.

If the doctor and nurse had applied the principles of TIC directly, they could have asked themselves: 'how could we make Hannah feel more safe during this intrusive procedure? Does she look like she feels comfortable in our presence? Are we paying attention to the relational space?' Knowledge of trauma would have ensured they could have collaborated on a quick plan to get through the procedure, agreeing that she could shut her eyes or stay quiet if she needed, as long as she indicated if she was not ok or needed them to stop. They could have enhanced trustworthiness by narrating the process of the procedure to Hannah as it occurred, giving clear explanations prior to inserting fingers or implements into her vagina, and actively sought consent. They could have given her choice by offering to close the curtain, asking where she wanted the nurse to stand, and letting Hannah indicate when she was ready to commence. They could have demonstrated empowerment by acknowledging the efforts Hannah employed to cope, by ensuring their focus was on her, and by checking what she needed to feel more comfortable. These small gestures are all indicators of trauma informed practice, but they do not equate to TIC. To be trauma informed would have required both the doctor and nurse to have approached this intervention with awareness of how common sexual violence is amongst women and the likelihood of this intervention being retraumatising. This would then guide all further actions, which would occur in attunement to the patient. If Hannah had not experienced trauma in her life, no harm would be done from the attentive approach and very little extra time would be added. As Hannah described, she had ways of coping and felt able to manage the procedure; thus, being trauma informed wouldn't have ensured that the procedure carried no risk of retraumatisation, but it would have improved Hannah's experience. In addition, the procedure may have been quicker and easier, saving them time, had they taken a few extra moments to ensure Hannah felt safe.

At the time I was writing this section of the book, I had coffee with some female friends who asked about the writing. I tell them the gist of Hannah's experience. The table comes alive with stories of upsetting or unsettling pap smears and intimate medical procedures. The table is lively as they describe things nurses and doctors have done or said, the violations they have felt. Speculums jammed in suddenly or too hard, comments about pubic hair, being left naked on the table, or getting in trouble for complaining about pain. After the buzz of stories settles, one of my friends sighs and says, 'It's funny how so many women go through these things and then we just pull our pants up, never speak of it again, and get on with our day as though we weren't just assaulted'. It is devastating to think of the care that we provide as akin to assault.

As in any circumstance, to be trauma informed when engaging with bodies is to be conscious of the possibility of shame and to do what you can to prevent it, while also being aware of possible signs that it is occurring in the moment. And to extend this sensitivity to conversations about bodies and to interactions involving any kind of scrutiny, examination, touching, or output of bodies (Box 10.3).

Box 10.3: Managing invasive procedures

- All forms of touch should be explained first ('this is what I am going to do and why'). This can still occur in emergencies or if people are not conscious.
- Consent should be sought, and when not possible, narration still provided ('I am just going to put my hand here to keep you still').
- Pre-arrange a signal to allow people to stop with ease ('just raise your hand if you want me to pause or stop').
- Avoid patronising names like 'honey' or 'darling'; these can be over-familiar or infantilise patients. These types of names are commonly used to put people at ease, but we don't know what context people may have heard them previously, and they can reinforce power and shame.
- Be conscious of who else is in the room or who else you are talking to while engaging in touch (as in, don't have a casual conversation with someone else while intimately touching someone else). Avoid talking as if the patient isn't there. I have seen nurses do this as a way to put people at ease, as though implying 'I am so unbothered by this that I can chat about my weekend with another nurse', but it can alienate people and lead to relational disconnection. The idea is to stay focused, attuned, and sensitive to the person.
- In the midst of invasive procedures, it is not the time to ask people questions about themselves. We may do this to try to distract them, but being asked about your plans for the weekend or your work is unsettling when you are already exposed and vulnerable.

- Offer choice wherever possible. This includes how procedures or examinations occur, as well as how you should act; for example, you can ask, 'would you prefer if we chat or stay quiet?'. Keep choices manageable and specific to minimise overwhelm.
- Observe verbal and non-verbal cues of patients' discomfort. (People who have experienced trauma may be overly compliant, so they do not want to tell you if it hurts. Look for muscle tension, curling toes, flinching, facial expressions, and so on.)
- Use kind words and assurance.
- Close doors or curtains entirely where possible and expose as little of a patient's body as is needed.
- Don't assume what people need or want – it is better to ask.
- Check if the person can do it for themselves, and if they can, and it is possible, let them.
- Remain conscious of boundaries. People may have been groomed or taught to ignore their own boundaries, and while we may be violating boundaries during procedures, we have an opportunity to narrate this, seek consent, and also maintain our own professional boundaries while doing so. This helps support safety.
- Avoid medicalised descriptions of bodies but stay professional. Consider how comments about any bodily related activity, output, or observation may be experienced by the person hearing it.
- If unsure, check in. ('How are you feeling about this? Is there anything we could do next time to make it better for you?')
- If you notice cues of triggering, dissociation, or distress, offer choice ('do you need to take a break?'), apologise if necessary ('I am sorry that this is uncomfortable'), and advise when it will end ('there is just one last bit left to do').
- Offer opportunities for debrief even if only momentarily ('did you have any questions you wanted to ask me about your body or that examination?').

Box 10.4: Clinical example: trauma informed care and dentists

Trauma informed dentists are a useful example of how to apply TIC to invasive procedures. Dentists do things to people in every appointment that are unpleasant, violating, painful, vulnerable, and shaming. They may be drilling or requiring you to have your mouth open for extended periods; they may be observing your dental care. There is a vulnerability about lying back and having your mouth violated that is distressing for many people, let alone people who have experienced trauma for whom it can be unbearable. But it would be a terrible thing if everyone with a history of trauma had to avoid dental care and therefore had teeth problems. This would be another injustice. And so, dentists are one group of health professionals really invested in how to work effectively with people who have experienced trauma, how to not make trauma worse for people, and how to make people feel safer in their chair, while still getting their dental work done. The work of being trauma informed is the work of the dentist; by that I mean that the assumption is not that patients manage themselves better or communicate their needs more (it's hard to communicate with your mouth open), and so trauma-informed dentists are focused on how they can establish and maintain safety.

There is something about the dental set-up that just clarifies some of the aspects of trauma informed care that can become confused in other settings. When verbal communication 'in the moment' is taken away, the dentist must set up the encounter for safety – discussing what people need, putting things in place to make people feel more comfortable, using distraction, and also setting up strategies that require no direct communication, for example, signals to use to take a break. When dental work is underway, it can be hard for people to express themselves, and they may be nervous to use the stop signal, so it remains the work of the dentist to notice slight shifts in the person's body and face and be responsive and sensitive to these cues. For example, they may notice the person curl their toes, tense their body, or crinkle their brow, and this should be enough for the dentist to pause and check in. Throughout the appointment, a trauma informed dentist is therefore focusing on what they are doing, while remaining attuned to what the person is needing, and if they are unable to do both of these, they usually have a dental assistant with them doing so. For some people, light sedation can help make the dental experience more manageable, but this does not equate to being trauma informed. Being sedated can make people feel more helpless and vulnerable. The loss of control or sense of being unable to defend oneself can be just as triggering as the procedure. It shouldn't be assumed what might make people feel safe. If we apply this idea to trauma informed nursing and midwifery, it makes it clear that trauma informed approaches don't have to change what care we deliver, just how we deliver it, with the onus of effort being on us to make sure we do what we can to make people feel safer in care.

Reference

O'Lynn, C., & Krautscheid, L. (2011). Original research: "How should I touch you?": A qualitative study of attitudes on intimate touch in nursing care. *American Journal of Nursing, 111*(3), 24–31. https://doi.org/10.1097/10.1097/01.NAJ.0000395237.83851.79

11 Conversations about trauma

To be trauma informed does not necessarily require talking about trauma; in fact, this usually takes time and trust. Being trauma informed is largely about considering what people might need, why they may be responding to you in certain ways, and considering interactions in the context of their lives. But it would also be incorrect to assume that you can be trauma informed without ever having conversations about trauma, sharing information, or knowledge about trauma. Talking directly about trauma can be one of the more 'scary' feeling components of trauma informed care as it requires us to demonstrate the ways that we are informed about trauma, not just to imply it through humanistic care. There is risk associated with this, risk of relational ruptures or discomfort, and risk of triggering occurring.

Asking about trauma

TIC can be delivered to anyone regardless of trauma history. However, to be aware of the specific impacts of trauma upon an individual, trauma also needs to be acknowledged. A point of contention in TIC is often when, how, and by whom a trauma history is specifically identified in healthcare delivery. There are a number of reasons why clinicians may be hesitant to ask about trauma, including time, lack of skills or specialist services, lack of clear role responsibilities, or fear of 'opening a can of worms'. Yet once we understand that trauma is prevalent, has significant effects on individuals, and also has impacts upon health, illness, and treatment, there becomes an imperative to ask about trauma in ways that keep people safe. Across studies, patients who have their trauma safely identified and responded to in health settings have significantly better health outcomes, fewer symptoms, and increased confidence in staff, suggesting that acknowledging and attending to trauma within existing therapeutic models can be therapeutic in itself.

Across studies with clinical populations, trauma history has been assessed without causing harm. For example, during the ACE Study (Felitti et al., 1998), in which 17,000 people participated in trauma questionnaires, no one was reportedly ever disturbed by the questions. If questions are asked at an appropriate time by an appropriate clinician, the 'success' of the interaction may be hampered by the clinician's confidence rather than the patient. Indeed, the most common reasons identified for not disclosing a history of trauma are feelings that the healthcare provider might not believe the story or might not be sensitive to the impact of trauma on current healthcare experiences.

Many TIC guides identify a need for universal screening for trauma in healthcare environments to ensure that trauma is accounted for and addressed in care. However,

DOI: 10.4324/9781003530770-14

asking about trauma requires sensitivity and skill and requires clarity of what pathways and responses are possible. As nurses and midwives, it is not always appropriate or timely to screen all patients for trauma histories. However, we need to feel confident to ask about experiences of trauma at appropriate times, and to respond safely to disclosures (Box 11.1).

Box 11.1: Asking about trauma

Best practice for screening for trauma history includes:

- the adaptation of screening practices to the setting (this means considering when is the best time within care for staff to be asking people about trauma and who is best placed to do so)
- ensuring that screening benefits the person being screened and the purpose is clear (this means considering how information about trauma is meaningfully incorporated into care planning and care delivery)
- avoiding repeated screening (this means considering how information about trauma is documented and shared amongst the team)
- ensuring ample staff training precedes screening (this means considering what skills, confidence, and knowledge staff require to be able to safely enquire about trauma and to be able to talk to people about trauma and its effects)

Using trauma screening tools

There is a difference between asking about people's experiences of trauma for the purpose of understanding, formulation, or providing effective care and screening for symptoms of a trauma disorder. It is important to know what the purpose of screening in your context is.

There are numerous available trauma screening tools, developed for various settings and populations. However, many trauma screening tools have been developed for research purposes, not for clinical purposes. This means they may try to categorise experiences across populations so that they can be reported and measured, by asking about exposure to predetermined events, without capturing the frequency, intensity, or duration, nor the associated dynamics, or protective factors. There are also many screening tools which screen solely for symptoms of PTSD. While these may be helpful in some circumstances, their routine use in healthcare does not equate to being trauma informed. Finding an appropriate tool and a safe enough process is important, alongside addressing the wider context and conversation that is needed to ensure we respond appropriately and safely.

In some settings, nurses and midwives routinely screen for trauma. For example, in maternity settings, nurses and midwives may screen all expectant parents for lifetime trauma to inform care planning. This can make the process normalised and unremarkable. After years of working in mental health services where asking about trauma was positioned as something the doctor or social worker should do, rather than nurses, I found it so interesting to work with midwives and early childhood nurses who were not only expected to screen but also to do so regularly with all patients, regardless of context. These experiences highlighted to me that it is possible for anyone to ask safely about trauma, and it is also possible for anyone to ask unsafely about trauma, regardless of the context. Nurses and midwives are often very well placed to ask people about trauma and how it may impact care, but to do so, we need support, resources, and opportunities to practise how to respond.

There is no best way to ask about trauma. How you ask will depend on your context and role. To be trauma informed in asking about trauma, it is usually helpful to give some warning about what you may ask, seek consent, and also give clarity about why you are asking, before you ask. For example, you might say 'the next couple of questions ask about things that have happened in your life, are you ok for me to ask you those now?' or you might say 'I try to ask everyone about experiences in their life that may be helpful for me to know about in ensuring I provide good care, is it ok if I ask you a few things about your life?'

Other questions you could try:

- *Is there anything that has happened in your life that it would be helpful for me to know?*
- *Lots of people I meet have experienced adversity or other related experiences in their lives that can impact care, would that be the case for you?*
- *We try to ask everyone who comes to our service about their lives so we can best tailor care, is it ok if I ask you some questions about things that may have happened to you?*

Often people who have experienced trauma may have also experienced unsupportive responses from people when they have tried to speak about these experiences. Silencing or disbelieving is a common response to disclosures. People can also feel silenced by other people's discomfort, disbelief, or horror. In healthcare contexts, people may disclose experiences of trauma for a variety of reasons. It is essential to always respond with sensitivity and care.

Responding to disclosures

Some people may find disclosure helpful and even cathartic. For others, it may not necessarily be something they want to do or are ready to do. People may not feel ready to talk about things that have happened to them for weeks, months, or years afterwards. Even if you hear people's trauma disclosures all the time in your work, your reaction to all disclosures is incredibly important. Trauma is so often woven with experiences of invalidation, shame, or being made to feel unimportant or inhuman in your needs. It can take bravery and hope to tell a healthcare professional about trauma. Responding in ways that demonstrate belief and validation is crucial to not re-enacting the dynamics of trauma.

In most clinical encounters, it is not necessary to ask a person for details of the event(s) which led to trauma or to explore in depth what happened to them. Instead, offer empathy and validation; for example, you might say 'that must have been very distressing/hard for you'. It is important to avoid blaming or shaming statements (such as 'why didn't you tell someone at the time' or 'why did they do that to you?'), which may reinforce guilt and self-blame. Often our role is validation and trust building, but also about identifying how experiences of trauma may be impacting health, illness, and care.

Sometimes our brains flood with all the actions that may be required if we know someone has a history of trauma or current experiences of trauma, but people are not usually telling us as they are expecting us to 'fix' it. They are telling us because it is an important part of their story or experience, and perhaps it is relevant to their current experience of illness, injury, or treatment or care. The priority is to listen, acknowledge, and identify links between past and present.

Often, we hear about the importance of letting people know we believe them. I have always been a bit unsure about saying overtly, 'I believe you'. We should always imply assumed belief. It arouses some irritation in me if people have said that specifically to me when I had no reason to doubt their belief. (Of course, you should believe me! Why wouldn't you believe me?!) But recently I had an experience of not being believed which made me think more deeply about the nuance of this. This is not a trauma story; it is an everyday annoyance story which reminded me of the importance of non-verbal communication of belief.

For years, I have had difficulties with a neighbour. The usual neighbour sorts of things around fences, trees, and rubbish bins. It has been a long-running problem, and the distress of it lies in the cumulative details over many years and the many little things that have caused harm. It's a little thing, but it does also cause me quite a lot of distress. I was telling my friend about the latest bit of the story recently and I noticed something in his face. He was looking at me and listening to me, but his eyes seemed to be almost smiling. There was a tiny suggestion of a smile or at least something in his expression that made me think 'He doesn't believe me'. As I recounted the details of the interaction, I could almost hear him thinking I was overreacting, or perhaps my neighbour hadn't meant it that way, or perhaps I had done something to deserve this, or perhaps I am making it up for the sake of the story. He didn't believe me. Or maybe he believed the facts, but he was questioning my emotional response, thinking it didn't seem 'that bad'. He didn't say anything, but I felt his disbelief.

This interaction reminded me of what it is like to tell someone a trauma experience and the attunement we feel to their eyes, their facial expression, their body language, their tone, and their vibe. We have many senses in our bodies. We have ways of feeling when it might rain, we have ways of feeling when we walk into a room and people are in the middle of a tense conversation, and we have a way of feeling when people don't believe us. So, as nurses and midwives, when people are telling us things that are distressing or important, the easiest way to address this is to just have a baseline approach of belief and to communicate this through our eyes, faces, and body language. We are not detectives; we don't need to gather evidence or prove something beyond a reasonable doubt. Our job is to care. In responding to disclosures, it actually usually doesn't matter what is objectively true or not. Sometimes people who are unwell or having anaesthetic or are distressed may make repeated disclosures of trauma that seem farcical. However, it is helpful to remember that the distress is real regardless of facts, and any dismissal of trauma disclosures should be handled with care and deep respect for the silencing and disbelief experienced by so many. There is very little point in arguing or disagreeing with anyone's disclosures, no matter how unlikely they seem. It may be that people are experiencing a blurring of past and present, and validation remains crucial. If needed, validation can occur alongside redirection or boundary setting.

In mental health nursing, we commonly hear stories that we are unsure if they happened in this reality or in an altered reality which the person is currently occupying due to psychosis, mania, or other reality-altering experiences. Sometimes we are sure that what the person is telling us did not happen because it is not possible. For example, we may be looking after someone on an inpatient unit who is very unwell, and they may yell at us that we raped them. While I know that people do get raped in hospitals, in this situation, let's assume we know it isn't true. This is highly distressing for everyone, but it is not uncommon. If I approach this with a baseline of belief, I believe that they are distressed, and I believe that they feel violated. I can still respond with care and empathy for the experience and the emotion and if possible I can get another nurse to take over care as a demonstration of respect for their distress and beliefs about me.

After we have validated people's experiences, we need to check what the person needs from us. People disclose for different reasons, and it may be helpful to understand what they want to happen next and to link back to the focus of your care. This may involve saying something like 'Would it be helpful to talk about how we can best support you while you are engaging with our service?', or 'Are there links between what you have told me and what is happening with your health?' Trauma can make us uncomfortable, and as a result, sometimes when people tell us something, we decide to never mention it again. This can be an avoidance or out of worry that we might say the wrong thing or upset them or make them feel uncomfortable. But as a healthcare professional, if a patient tells us about trauma in their lives, it is nearly always necessary to follow up on the conversation. It may even just be 'how are you feeling about what we spoke about earlier?'

Part of the shame and blame of trauma experiences is the way that they are minimised in our minds. Minimising or downplaying events may occur as part of a survival strategy (as in, we tell ourselves it wasn't that bad to enable us to keep going) or it may be an internalised belief fostered by the perpetrator of harm. Often, part of the dynamic of trauma that occurs interpersonally is that the perpetrator denies that their actions are harmful. This is confusing and part of the control and manipulation that forms part of many relational traumas. We may also blame ourselves for not having stopped something from happening, or for having consented to parts of things but not all of things, or for having maintained relationships with people who have hurt us. When traumas are environmental or don't involve another human, we may tell ourselves that it wasn't as bad as it could have been, or that others had it worse than we did. It may also be that what happened wasn't 'that bad', but what could have happened or what didn't happen is what has led to trauma. This makes sense but can be hard to articulate or understand. For example, in experiences of neglect, it may be that a child missed out on love, delight, play, vitality, protection, and so on. From one perspective, nothing 'bad' might have happened, but so much hurt and trauma is created in the gaps and missing bits. This can also be true when things nearly happen. I have met people deeply traumatised by near misses or imagined losses. While one part of the brain seems unable to distinguish between things that didn't happen and things that might, another part of the brain is set on telling us how unimportant and irrelevant that feeling is. The brain is a contradictory and complex organ. It is therefore crucial that we validate and hold space for the importance of these experiences. People may rush or brush over them in the telling of things or talk about them with big emotion and then invalidate themselves ('it's silly' or 'it doesn't matter'). Just circling back and saying how hard that must have been for them and that it makes sense that they feel upset can be very powerful.

Sometimes we need to help people pace their disclosures of trauma to avoid an internal avalanche of emotion. An example I can think of is, years ago I was interviewing a doctor about their understanding of trauma and the questions must have activated her own trauma response. All of a sudden, stories of trauma were spilling out of her; she was telling me about children who had been abused, her own experiences of violence, and clients she had cared for. The stories overlapped and the telling felt out of control. Her eyes were fixed on me but also vacant. I felt I needed to help her stop. I remember first tuning into my own body, desperately trying to consider how to create stillness and mindful presence, and then looking for any moment I could intercept. I did so suddenly, and as gently as I could, by saying her name when she took a breath. She looked at me and paused, and I said something like 'I can hear you have witnessed *a lot* of pain'. This was an intentional statement. I wanted her to hear that it felt like *a lot*. I wanted her to feel seen – that I noticed how much she was carrying. I wanted to name it pain. And I also wanted to give her a chance to stop, or to interrupt the flow of a river she seemed to be flowing down. I remember she paused, and her gaze returned; she apologised. We sat in silence for a few moments, and the moment passed.

In general, a person needs to be believed, listened to, and have a sense that it is a good thing they have told you. They should be given time and space to make their own decisions about next steps. During this process, keep in mind that a sense of agency and control is key to trauma recovery (Box 11.2).

Box 11.2: Responding to disclosures of trauma

- Thank people for telling you. To be listened to and experiences validated can be powerful.
- You do not need to ask questions or details. It is not your role to piece together all aspects of events or to ensure disclosures are accurate.
- You can listen without judgement and validate emotion without knowing details. At times, people feel compelled to tell you details for their own reasons. It can be helpful to support them to pace the disclosure by letting them know you believe them and that they only need to share what they feel comfortable sharing.
- If they are distressed or dysregulated when sharing details, you may want to encourage them to slow down or take a break.
- Manage your own reactions. Sometimes hearing about trauma can be shocking and you may want to acknowledge the shock you feel; however, visible shock or distress can trigger shame in the person telling you the experience.
- Reacting is ok, but it shouldn't dominate the interaction. It can be helpful to ask people who else they have told to understand the wider context of disclosure and previous responses.
- You may not feel like the most skilled or confident person to respond to their disclosure (or you may lack time), in which case it is important to validate and acknowledge as well as offering further support from an experienced person.
- It is important to see what they need to feel safe right now and beyond, including letting them know what you will do with the information they have shared.
- It may be helpful to ask people how their experiences of trauma impact their current circumstances and whether there is anything that may assist them to feel safer in care.
- If you are unsure what support is available, it is ok to let them know that you will get back to them with additional support and resources (just make sure that you do).

Recognising resistance

There are conflicts in asking people who have experienced trauma to tell us about the events that harmed them. If we just focus on the trauma and the acts of harm, we can risk re-enacting dynamics of trauma, blaming the person who experienced the events, or reinforcing shame. Within all experiences of trauma, there is resistance. Asking about trauma to identify ways our care may be triggering for people should also be balanced by asking about how people have managed to survive times of fear and horror, as this will also inform our understanding of how to help them stay safe. Acts of resistance usually don't stop trauma occurring and shouldn't be overly romanticised or positioned as heroic. It is also important to focus on what the person views as resistance, as not all acts are resistance. Questions like 'how did you manage to survive?' or 'what helped you to get through that?' can help to draw out people's strengths and acts. Identifying what happened to people and how they got through it and continue to survive is not about identifying symptoms of trauma or vulnerability but about recognizing people's experiences and refocusing on their humanity. Often when you ask people about their experiences and how they got through them, they may shrug or say 'I don't know'. This gives you an opportunity together to reflect on what strengths the person may have that they haven't realised.

Box 11.3: Clinical example: recognising resistance

Jaya is a 24-year-old woman who presented to an emergency department following an unintentional overdose of prescription pain medications. She was stabilised but admitted overnight for monitoring of her kidney function. On the nephrology ward, she is cared for by Troy, a Registered Nurse. Over Troy's morning shift, he has built rapport with Jaya and tried to demonstrate respect, dignity, and trust by the way he speaks with her, his responsiveness to her needs, and his consistent warm and non-judgmental attitude. Jaya has already been asked a lot of questions in the emergency department about why she took the medications, why she had the medications, and the events. Jaya explained to the admitting doctor that she started taking pain medications after a minor medical procedure last year and found the tablets made her feel numb. Recently, her stepfather died, and she had started taking the tablets again to cope. Prior to her admission, she had got confused and taken too many. She asked her flatmate to bring her to the hospital as a precaution. Troy has been asked to gather a bit more information in the lead up to her discharge. Troy asks Jaya if its ok if he asks her some questions about the things that led up to her admission. When she agrees, he ensures privacy, sits down, and begins.

Troy:	*Maybe if we start with me just going over what I know from your notes and you letting me know if its correct. I understand that your stepfather recently died which must have been really upsetting, and that is what led to you starting to take the pain medications that you still had from your procedure last year. I also understand from the notes that you hadn't meant to take so many and had no intention to overdose. Is that all correct? Is there anything I haven't got right?*
Jaya:	*I guess it's mostly correct.*
Troy:	*When you say 'mostly correct', are there any bits you want to go over? I can make sure to update the notes if any of that doesn't feel right.*

Jaya:	*I think just how you said I was feeling isn't exactly what I told the doctor. I mean, yes my stepfather died but I actually wasn't upset about that. I didn't take the tablets because I was sad.*
Troy:	*Oh … ok, I'm sorry, I think I just read what he had written and assumed you were upset. I'm sorry I assumed that. Is it ok if I ask you some questions about your stepfather and how you did feel when he died?*
Jaya:	*yeah*
Troy:	*What was your relationship like with your stepfather?*
Jaya:	*He wasn't a nice man. Our relationship wasn't good.*
Troy:	*Ok, got it, he wasn't nice and your relationship wasn't good. Can you tell me anything more about that?*
Jaya:	*He was really violent actually. He used to beat my mum, me and my sister. Ever since we were small until I left home. To be honest, I am glad he's dead.*
Troy:	*Gosh. I'm sorry to hear that. That sounds like a lot to go through. How did you manage to get through your childhood?*
Jaya:	*I don't know … what choice did I have?*
Troy:	*I can imagine you were quite stuck. Was there anything you remember doing in the very hard moments to get through?*
Jaya:	(thinks for awhile, then speaks slowly) *Well … I sort of learned how not to feel anything. I had this way of disappearing in my mind. Then it was like I wasn't there and he couldn't hurt me.*
Troy:	*Incredible. [pauses]. How did you figure out how to do that?*
Jaya:	*I don't know. I used to try to protect my sister. So, I would try to distract him, which meant I always copped it. So I needed some way to escape I guess.*
Troy:	*It's a pretty great strategy to protect your sister, even if it then harmed you.*
Jaya:	*I guess.*
Troy:	*Do you still sometimes disappear with your mind?*
Jaya:	*Only if I take too many pain medications! I mean … not so much. Sometimes I wish I could I guess. I mostly don't think about the past, but when he died I had to think about it. Everyone at his funeral was saying nice things about him and I felt so angry and I would have liked to escape. I think the medication helped with that.*
Troy:	*That makes sense. You had a way to cope with what happened to try to keep you and your sister safe. It makes sense that the medication gave you a shortcut to try to do that again.*
Jaya:	*True … Although it didn't really keep me safe this time as now I'm here.*
Troy:	*Maybe we could talk a bit more with the team about other ways to keep you safe when you go home, so that you aren't taking medication you don't need but also so you don't feel trapped with your thoughts and emotions.*

Nurses and midwives work in diverse settings, so it may be that this interaction in Box 11.3 doesn't fit with your context and how much time or opportunity you have to talk with people about their experiences. However, in this interaction, a pretty brief conversation was woven into the course of usual discharge planning. Troy attended to power by seeking consent, sitting down, and ensuring privacy (Box 11.4).

Box 11.4: Reflections on Troy's response to Jaya's disclosure

- Troy attended to power by seeking consent, sitting down, and ensuring privacy.
- He shared his power with Jaya right from the start by telling her the information he had from her notes. This is an act of transparency but also ensures people have control over what is written and shared about them.
- Troy managed to identify Jaya's experiences of trauma, as well as recognising her capacity to cope and survive. He did this through staying focused on her and what she did, rather than by focusing on details of the violence or her stepfather.
- Troy drew out acts of resistance in amongst trauma. Witnessing these and noticing them can have a profound impact upon people's sense of self – reinforcing the ways they have survived rather than the things that happened.
- He didn't ask her to relive or share traumatic details. It would have been easy for him to ask more questions about the violence, how often it occurred, and how severe it was. But this would have risked opening up a larger conversation than he had time or skills to manage safely. Instead, his response to her disclosure stayed focused on her and how she coped.
- He wasn't pitying or condescending. Sometimes our shock and horror or distress at peoples' experiences, even when well intentioned, can reinforce shame.
- He stayed focused on the present, linking events she shared from the past with what was happening right now. This kept her safer and ensured he stayed within the scope of his role.
- He offered hope by implying there are things that could be done to try to help her feel and be safe.
- He validated that her behaviour and coping strategies made sense and that her actions had the intended purpose of keeping her sister and herself safe. This is the act of witnessing, validating, and ensuring the person's agency is recognised.
- He brought others into the conversation by mentioning the wider team to break down a sense of secrecy or shame.

Talking directly about trauma

Understanding of trauma should inform how we interact with people, how we understand their experiences, and how we manage ourselves. But it should not be secret information that we don't share with the person accessing care if it is appropriate to do so. This relates to power. There is a power imbalance in healthcare in part because we hold and share information about people, being trauma informed shouldn't add to this. Of course, this doesn't mean telling people 'I think you have trauma' or 'You are reacting this way because of trauma'. It might mean introducing the idea of trauma gently or giving people opportunities to think about trauma. It is important to ensure you have time and are in a physically safe feeling space to talk directly about trauma. It is also important to introduce the topic in ways that won't make people feel ambushed. This means giving people a choice about whether they want information or are interested in hearing about your understanding of trauma. It also means that you keep an open mind about how the person makes sense of their own experiences and don't assume that a trauma lens is helpful to everyone.

One aspect of conversations about trauma is helping people to hold those parts of their lives as part of their story but to also separate them even a tiny bit from themselves. I often say to people that I don't know the answers and I don't always know anything that will help but that it can be helpful to lay out all the bits together and just talk about them and look at them. In my mind, I imagine it like a pocket full of rocks that people carry around, and for a brief period they pass some of the rocks to me. Together we lay them out and look at them, think about them, admire them, acknowledge them, and then carefully gather them back into the pocket. In separating things (whether they be difficult memories, trauma experiences, or shame parts) from our full self and imagining them as either separate parts of us or external things all together that we carry, things become more manageable. How we make this distinction can often be quite subtle. For example, someone might say 'I just feel so embarrassed', and we could reply 'do you think we could talk more about the part of you that feels that way?' or someone could say 'I've felt like this my whole life' and we might say 'are there times or even moments where you have felt differently?' or someone might say 'I hate that I do that' and we might say 'do you think it has served a purpose for you at some points in your life?' These are just slight reframes that allow for the idea of complexity and contradiction; that the person is not what has happened to them and that how they respond to things is not flawed but perhaps an adaptation to adversity.

Safe enough storytelling

How much detail should be shared about traumatic events is highly contextual. If you are a nurse in an emergency department, a sexual health clinic, or a service where you are asking about violence or abuse, you need to be prepared to sit with all the details. This will likely include hearing about acts, injuries, or events that are shocking. This will involve you managing your own reactions to minimise seeming shocked, over-whelmed, or distressed. So often I have heard survivors talk of the burden it places on them if the person they are trying to tell the story to can't hold it. 'How do you think it is for me who lived it?' a woman said to me recently when talking about how a health-care worker had asked her to stop while she was sharing her story.

There are, however, times when it is important for there to be more safety within the storytelling. For example, if someone at a new parents' group starts talking about their child-hood abuse in detail, it may be highly distressing for the other participants. Or if someone is sharing the details with a whole multidisciplinary team in a forum where, perhaps later, they may feel shame or distress. It is also an issue encountered often in education sessions or research settings. People may either get activated in their memory and start sharing in depth, or they may be trying to justify or explain something, or they may be offering contributions that they think you need. It can be very difficult when you have lived through trauma to always know what is 'appropriate' or acceptable to share in what circumstances.

As nurses and midwives, we need to give people a bit of a signpost of what is expected. For example, if I am asking someone about their past in a clinical context, I need to be open to hearing as much as they share, so I might say something like 'Please tell me as many details as you feel comfortable sharing'. If they express concern that I may find the details distressing, this is a good time to use the 'I'm a nurse (or a midwife) and I spend a lot of time with people in vulnerable situations. I may be upset imagining that this happened to you but it will not be too much for me to hear'. Often people who have experienced trauma have been told or picked up messages that they are 'too much' or that it is 'too much' for other people to cope with. Trauma overwhelms our capacity to cope; therefore, trauma is always 'too much'. But the person who experienced it or who is telling the story is never too much. If you do find it 'too much' to hear, this is important for you to seek support with afterwards. Vicarious trauma also occurs when we are being overwhelmed by other people's stories. It isn't helpful to assume we can absorb everything and not be impacted.

In a healthcare context, we need to set clear boundaries and then guide people through them, minimising shame. This means if it is a situation where we need just a certain level of detail but not all of the details, it is helpful to be explicit about that. You might say, 'I am just going to ask you a few details about what happened, but at this stage there is no need to include all of the details. Perhaps if you can just tell me the events and then once we get you sorted out, we can talk more about the details.' However, even this can be too vague. Recently, I facilitated some group consultations with women who have experienced domestic and family violence. They were all there because of their lived experiences of violence, and we wanted them to reflect on these experiences in developing a resource. How to best navigate safe storytelling in such a context is a challenge. But it is a challenge for us as facilitators, not the participants. They turn up and share their experiences as asked. But I was conscious of the potential for the details of violence to be triggering for participants or perhaps even for me. After a few introduction attempts that asked people to be considerate of the group and only share things they feel comfortable with, I realised we had to be much more specific. By the final group, the introduction included 'We are all here because we are willing to talk about and hear about each other's experiences which involve violence. However, please try to minimise including details of particularly distressing acts or injuries, particularly those involving children. If you start sharing a lot about violence, we might gently interrupt you by saying your name. This can feel jarring. If this does happen, we will also follow up with you after the session to check in'. This was my attempt to make the storytelling within the space safe-enough. It lets people know the clear boundary of what is ok and less ok and also sets up a plan for interruption, as sometimes when people start talking, you can see the moment that they lose control over themselves. The words start pouring out and they are back in that moment. I wanted them to know that they may hear their name, and this may bring them back to the present and give them a few moments to regroup.

These words aren't perfect and will not ensure every group or interaction goes smoothly, but part of being trauma informed is giving people a clear expectation upfront of what is expected. This minimises shame and fear and also keeps us and our patients safe. Such guidance is also relevant in busy clinic situations or shared ward rooms where you might say, 'Because this isn't a private space/or we don't have much time together, I want to ask you a few questions and if you can just share…'. It is also relevant in home visits if there are children or other family members nearby where you might say something like: 'Because your child is here, I won't ask you to go into any detail about the events and there may be also a few things I ask you to just pause and tell me a bit later in the appointment when we are on our own'. The key thing here is that this is someone's experience and life and it isn't for them to censor it for our benefit. However, it is helpful for us to leverage our healthcare worker power as nurses and midwives by managing the space prior to asking or opening up a conversation.

Empathic interrupting

Things can also catch you off guard. Someone may just launch into a story unexpectedly in a space which feels not great for you (such as with a child present or in a multi bed hospital unit).

Empathic interrupting is a way to manage the intensity or content that someone is telling you or to slow down a story so you can support the person to regulate their distress and arousal. We are often taught that all interrupting is rude, but sometimes interrupting is an act of care when we see danger or risk. For example, if someone drops something while they are walking and talking to their friend, we will interrupt to let them know. If my friend was chatting while we walked and they didn't see a car coming, I would interrupt them to keep them safe. I may touch their arm while I interrupt or I might apologise or help them reorient afterwards, but I would prioritize safety. There are times when it is also important to interrupt patients. In a study about doctors interrupting patients, Mauksch (2017) identified a strategy for interrupting in empathic ways. He calls it 'The Triple E'. The first 'E' is *excuse* yourself. You might say 'I'm sorry to interrupt' or you might say 'Can I just stop you for a moment?' This step acknowledges the socialised 'insensitivity' of your interruption. The second 'E' is *empathise*. This requires you to directly empathise with what the person is saying at the point of interruption. Acknowledging the specific thing the person is saying will let them know that you are listening and decrease the chance of them feeling shamed. You might say, 'what you are telling me about what happened that day is really important', or you might say, 'The pain you are describing sounds really overwhelming'. The third 'E' is *explain*. This requires you to explain why you interrupted. Giving a transparent reason will help the person stay engaged rather than feeling invalidated or shamed. You might say, 'I just want to make sure I understand what you were just saying first', or you might say, 'I want to make sure that you feel like you want to tell me all of this right now'.

In the context of a trauma story, you need to be careful but using Mauksch's EEE approach is a good way to reorient the person to what is happening in this immediate moment (Box 11.5).

Box 11.5: Clinical example of empathic interrupting

Lola is talking to her midwife, Chandi, answering questions as part of her psychosocial assessment at her booking appointment. Chandi asks Lola if she has a history of domestic violence and Lola hesitates. She says no. Chandi nods. Lola then says, 'Actually, maybe yes' and starts to describe her experiences in a past relationship in her early twenties. She starts to talk rapidly, expressing uncertainty and losing cohesion. She says, 'I mean it was violence in the sense that I understand it now, but I didn't understand it as that then'. Chandi nods and moves her hand to tick yes on the form. Lola keeps going: 'He used to trick me into doing things you know. Like is that violence? I felt like I had to. I felt scared. But sometimes I'm not sure if I was just young. Like sometimes he would...' Chandi has a sense that Lola is experiencing re-enactments. Her eyes are darting around the room and she is wringing her hands. Chandi feels uneasy. She decides to interrupt. She says, 'Lola, I'm sorry to cut you off (e). What you are telling me about these experiences is really important (e). But I want you to know that you don't need to explain to me if you don't want to (e)'. Lola meets Chandi's eyes and nods. It gives Chandi a chance to continue. She explains why they ask these questions and how they can inform the way they deliver care. She explains her understanding of violence as personal and that the dynamics of control can often mean people don't realise it is violence straight away. She explains that it is ok for her to tick yes on the form if Lola wants her to, without needing to know or judge exactly what happened.

In Box 11.5, Chandi wanted to interrupt so she could clarify the intent of the question and ensure Lola didn't share more than she wanted to. She was also likely concerned about the interaction getting derailed from its clinical intent, and that is also a legitimate reason to interrupt. Mauksch warns that 'Interruption is a sharp knife' (p. 1022). This is a timely warning in the context of being shame sensitive. Interruptions should always be done respectfully and with transparency. A truthful explanation goes a long way; for example, people usually don't mind being told how much time or resources you have, or what your priorities are for the time you have; they may rather an explanation than just having a sense of you being rushed or bothered. Knowing when to interrupt is a balance of care, instinct, and noticing, and we don't always get it right.

References

Felitti, V. J., Anda, R. F., Nordenberg, D., Williamson, D. F., Spitz, A. M., Edwards, V., Koss, M. P., & Marks, J. S. (1998). Relationship of childhood abuse and household dysfunction to many of the leading causes of death in adults. *American Journal of Preventive Medicine, 14*(4), 245–258. https://doi.org/10.1016/S0749-3797(98)00017-8

Mauksch, L. B. (2017). Questioning a taboo: Physicians' interruptions during interactions with patients. *JAMA, 317*(10), 1021. https://doi.org/10.1001/jama.2016.16068

12 Lifespan considerations for trauma informed practice

People change over their life course. Development is a dynamic interaction that occurs between people and their environment, leading to changes in understanding of self, priorities, relationships, behaviour, and activities. Trauma impacts differ across the lifespan, but so does how we understand it. As nurses and midwives, we adapt our care to the needs of people at different stages of the lifespan, and in doing so need to consider the unique ways that knowledge of trauma can inform this care.

Trauma informed perinatal care

The perinatal period encompasses conception to the first year after birth. The perinatal period is a time of significant change. For parents, it can be a time of reflection on self and life, a time of potential or actual loss of control, and can also be the time that people engage with health services heavily for the first time and receive intrusive observations and interventions.

Pregnancy can impact people who have experienced trauma in unexpected ways. It can interrupt existing coping mechanisms people use to minimise the effects of trauma upon their lives (such as exercise, drinking, or excessive working), past experiences can be activated through changing bodies and processes, or new trauma can be caused through the process of pregnancy and birth. Trauma is linked to adverse physiological experiences which impact the developing or new infant through cortisol levels, reduced foetal growth, preterm birth, interventional births, low birthweight, and postpartum distress and depression for parents. However, birth and parenting can also be a powerful healing experience for many people who have experienced trauma and infants can thrive despite trauma within family units.

Parents presenting for pregnancy or birthing care may not directly recognise or identify trauma. Some may actively try to not focus on the past during a future-focussed time. I have seen many people who have seen pregnancy as an opportunity to change their lives or try to do or be 'better' for their infant than anyone was for them. People may also be acutely concerned about the possible impacts of trauma or stress upon their baby, or their capacity to parent. As such, a strengths-based approach is important. The sensitivity of this time is also important as people may respond unexpectedly or disjointedly to questions about their lives and be highly sensitive to feelings of shame or judgement. Nurses and midwives being sensitive, aware, and confident in thinking about and talking about trauma is crucial.

Triggering of trauma during the perinatal period may mean that people display hypersensitivity, disproportionate distress, or experiences of sadness, fear, pain, anger, and shame. This can occur as it can in any healthcare encounter, as a result of power

DOI: 10.4324/9781003530770-15

differentials, clinical settings, loss of control, and busy clinicians, but it is also more likely due to reminiscent bodily experiences. Trauma can be replicated through intrusive interventions, as well as a sense of someone else having control of your body, violation, objectification, powerlessness, or vulnerability. Sometimes the triggering of trauma is also woven into the experience of pregnancy itself. When trauma has occurred within attachment relationships, it can be triggered during pregnancy due to activation of the attachment system. I have seen many pregnant people highly distressed by this experience as it can often occur beneath consciousness and feel like something is very wrong.

Attachment processes begin prenatally through physical, kinaesthetic, and intellectual awareness of the infant. The sensation of the baby, the shared physicality and perception of the baby, and thoughts and hopes for the baby all contribute to attachment. Many people experience complex emotional responses during pregnancy, both positive and negative, and trauma can be woven through these. Emotions can include tenderness and preoccupation, as well as fear, avoidance, anger, ambivalence, or sadness. Parents may not link these emotions to attachment and may instead feel shame or confusion about what they are feeling when everyone assumes it is a happy or joyful time. It is possible to explore these responses through gentle questions about what the person is doing to prepare for the baby, how they are imagining themselves as a parent, and how they are feeling about the baby. While these questions are common in pregnancy care, trauma sensitivity means that nurses and midwives are intentional in their approach and attuned not just to the responses, but the way the stories are told, the emotions present, and the parents' affect (Box 12.1).

Box 12.1: Trauma woven into attachment experiences

Suzanne is a client I worked with for perinatal anxiety when pregnant with her first baby. She describes herself as 'always an anxious person'. She has a highly successful and stressful job. Her pregnancy is a long-awaited IVF pregnancy, and she is happy to be pregnant. However, in mid-pregnancy she starts experiencing intrusive thoughts of harm to her body from her baby. She experiences her baby as intrusive and his movements make her feel physically sick. She has a sense of 'being abused' by him and feels powerless. She is teary when talking about this. At her midwifery appointment, when she is asked about her childhood, she describes medical trauma as a child from a painful investigation. Since this time, she has felt anxious about hospitals; she feels she may lose control in hospitals and her body won't be hers. She describes her parents as 'controlling', her mother through intrusion into her privacy and her father through power and threats. She moved to the other side of the world as she felt it was the only way to have control over her own life. She loves her baby, but she always imagined she would have a daughter, and she feels confused by her emotions towards her unborn son. She is ashamed of the complex emotions and feels people can't understand.

In being able to talk about these experiences, she reduces shame and starts to make links between the past, the triggering of relational trauma, and the fear of loss of bodily control she feels. She begins to understand some of the emotions she has towards her son. It doesn't take away the thoughts, but it does take away some of the emotions attached to them and it gives her a way to make sense of things that previously felt shaming and scary.

For parents with knowledge and awareness of their own attachment backgrounds, particularly those involving trauma, they may worry overtly about replicating experiences. This can lead to parents expressing worry, preoccupation with excessive preparation, and expectation. Alongside these experiences of preoccupying anxiety, others may feel 'numb', with daydreams or nightmares of running away or abandoning their baby, leading to shame and fear. Attachment experiences during pregnancy differ from early parenting attachment experiences as there are less opportunities for reciprocation because the baby isn't yet present and mirroring the experience. Without reciprocity during pregnancy, anxiety may embed as a mechanism of responding to experiences of fear and loss of control. Supporting understanding of how these unexpected experiences may relate to the process of attachment itself, rather than feelings about the infant directly, can be a critical task for nurses and midwives. While these experiences are not uncommon, they create opportunities for nurses and midwives to support understanding and awareness of the attachment process, within conversations, normalising how past experiences can influence the present. This benefits the parent but also the infant.

A key task of the perinatal period is also birth. Birth can trigger activation of trauma memories and responses. While we may easily think about how sexual traumas could relate to birth, the vulnerability and loss of control during birth can seemingly activate all kinds of traumas. Birth itself can also be traumatic if it is long, goes unexpectedly, leads to overwhelming pain, injury, or fear. The shock of birth not meeting expectations can also be traumatic in ways that people outside of midwifery or perinatal care may not appreciate.

Trauma informed birth care planning

Birth care planning can be an important component of trauma informed care during the perinatal period. This type of planning differs from planning about the type of birth you want. This is about the type of care people need during experiences of birth, in the context of trauma (Box 12.2).

Box 12.2: Clinical example of a trauma informed birth care plan

The patient has a history of childhood sexual abuse.

Environment

Patient is concerned about privacy and losing control of her body. Where possible, please provide a blanket to hold and ensure her body is covered when undertaking examinations.

Patient plans to be supported by her sister throughout labour and delivery. Her sister will provide verbal reassurance and advocacy.

Communication

Patient would like all procedures to be explained in simple, clear language to her and her sister, and where possible, steps to be narrated as procedures are undertaken. Please ask for consent before any physical contact or procedure. Patient often experiences dissociation during bodily examinations. This may mean she is unable to communicate clearly. Sister may answer on her behalf if this occurs.

Physical comfort

Patient is concerned about experiencing pain and discomfort in her lower body as this can be a trigger. She would prefer early use of an epidural or other pain management if possible. Patient would prefer not to lie on her back throughout delivery.

Emotional support

Patient is terrified of feeling helpless and finds verbal support reassuring. She finds the statement 'You are ok, you are safe' reassuring. Patient identifies trauma triggers as the smell of cleaning products and unexpected physical touch. Where these can't be avoided, please provide reassurance and remind her to engage her usual coping strategies.

Interventions

Patient would prefer minimal internal examinations unless necessary. Patient would prefer not to watch as her baby is born.

Post-birth care

Patient plans to breastfeed but is nervous about the sensation. Please provide support around initial breast attachment. Please offer a debriefing session in the days after delivery if required.

Such plans are not about dictating care; they are a nursing and midwifery care plan and a way of handing over collaborative strategies for managing trauma in the context of birth. The plan is important, but the process of making the plan is equally important as it creates a sense of control and action amongst fear.

Trauma informed care with infants

Trauma can occur at any age, including prior to verbal development or memory. Infants and neonates can likely experience trauma without knowing. In these early stages of life, the brain's most primitive role is to promote survival, with any experience that poses a perceived or actual threat to survival triggering a series of survival mechanisms. The amygdala, which plays a key role in trauma responses, is thought to be functional from about 23 weeks of gestation. This does not mean that any event of stress will be traumatic, but it means that stressful or life-threatening events (including birth, neonatal illness, or attachment disruptions) can become potentially traumatic events. Experiences of persistent lack of soothing or care can also be experienced as life-threatening for infants.

Infant trauma has been studied in Neonatal Intensive Care Units (NICU). The context of the NICU is one of constant noise, light, monitoring, and activity to ensure the survival and well-being of neonates. Much work has been done to make the environments of NICUs more conducive to soothing and neuroprotection, for example, through dimmed lighting, kangaroo care, single rooms, and comfort items. However, the experience that neonates go through in the NICU can equate to a unique form of trauma named 'Infant Medical trauma' (D'Agata et al., 2016), linked to stress, pain, and parental separation. NICU is, however, also essential to survival. We don't need to know if it is or isn't traumatic to be trauma informed; we can just respond as nurses and midwives to infants and caregivers who are under stress in ways that try to minimise the impacts, by being responsive, sensitive, consistent, and supportive of attachment. Infants can cope with traumatic events if they have responsive and sensitive caregiving most of the time.

The importance of attachment

Attachment refers to relationships and bonds (particularly long-term) between people, commencing with those between a caregiver and infant. Humans need to 'attach' to other humans for survival. Secure attachments support emotional regulation, reduce fear, and help infants develop the processes required for attunement to the needs of other people, as well as expression of their own needs, self-understanding, and empathy. When infants feel safe in their relationships with their caregivers, they trust their needs will be met and they will be cared for, they learn how to regulate their own emotions, and slowly they also learn about the emotional worlds of others. Insecure attachments, or those where an infant cannot rely on an adult to respond to their needs consistently in times of stress, can interrupt development and lead to challenges with self-soothing, managing emotions, and engaging in reciprocal relationships.

Infants are born unable to manage their own emotions, thoughts, or behaviours. They rely on adults to cuddle them, rock them to sleep, comfort them in distress, delight in them, and teach them to interact and play. They reach for things, and we smile in delight They smile at us, and we smile back. When they are sad, we make soft noises, hold them close, and pat or rock them. Through these repeated acts, they slowly learn to do it themselves. They learn to settle themselves to sleep, they learn to play and distract themselves, they learn that when they are sad and need help, someone will come and soothe them, they learn that they are loveable, and within this context, they slowly start to manage their own needs.

Trauma in these relationships does not occur from occasional or infrequent insensitivities, but from abrupt separation, or a repeated lack of care or attention. Traumas of infancy can also result from caregiver emotional dysregulation (Lyons–Ruth et al., 2006) woven into the everyday interactions between caregiver and infants. These dynamics can be hard to recognise as they may not appear as overt harm or neglect; they are important for nurses and midwives to be aware of as there is a lot of evidence to suggest that subtle, sustained traumatic dynamics during infancy lead to physiologic consequences similar to overt threat events.

Attachment relationships are pivotal to so many relational traumas and infant and child experiences. The most important nursing and midwifery trauma informed intervention during infancy is supporting parent/caregiver and infant attachment through the therapeutic relationship. Our presence in the relationship models reflective functioning by regulating ourselves so we can support parents, and supporting the regulation of parents, so they can support infants. Our role is to help identify the emotional states of parents and infants and to support sensitivity and responsiveness to what might be happening in the inner world of the infant.

Trauma informed care with children

Children may experience trauma from events in their homes, their communities, their environment, or exposure to external events. Trauma that occurs within families can be related to physical, emotional, or sexual abuse, neglect, exposure to domestic and family violence, or intergenerational trauma. Children are also vulnerable to harm perpetrated by peers, teachers, or other adults, as well as bullying, poverty, war, displacement, climate change, unsafe living conditions, loss of family members, parental incarceration, parental drug use, parental mental illness, out of home care, intrusive medical procedures, or illness. While many causes of childhood trauma are overt acts of violence or exposure to distressing circumstances or threats, the reliance of children upon adults to meet their needs means that they are also highly vulnerable to trauma arising from neglect. Trauma in childhood is relevant to context. This means that in some cultures, children are expected to be far more independent at earlier ages. It does not mean that children are less impacted by traumatic things, but rather, what is considered traumatic may differ.

Providing trauma informed care for children involves understanding and addressing the impact of trauma on their physical and emotional well-being. Children may not be able to tell us what has happened to them, and we shouldn't push them to put words to it. It may come out in play or non-verbal ways, or not at all. They may still be in survival dynamics of safe/unsafe or worried about causing distress to their parents or families.

Beyond child protection responsibilities to identify and intervene when there is active trauma, our responsibility as nurses and midwives lies in the present moment. In the present moment, we can be safe and trustworthy, we can demonstrate how we perceive their importance and power, we can reflect our delight in them back to them, and we can provide them with ways and opportunities to express themselves. Providing care to children in ways that are trauma informed also requires us to role model safe relationships. This includes narrating the process of consent and touch with children, actively attending to privacy and self-agency, and redirecting any attempts to blur boundaries. For brief periods of time we take on a role as a trusted figure with children in our care which requires modelling relational and attachment behaviours of responsiveness and sensitivity to their needs, reinforcing their developing sense of self through direct and specific reflections (e.g. 'you seem to be a very smart person, you notice everything' or 'Thank you so much for remembering that about me, that's very kind'), and providing words to their experiences and emotions ('It looks like you are sad, do you feel sad?'). Children are often shamed in adult conversations about them, so it is important to protect their agency and personhood in the ways we talk to them and about them.

Children are highly connected and attuned to their families. Excluding when there are child protection concerns related to the family unit, we need to engage families and work alongside families and not compromise the loyalty all children feel to their parents. We can be curious about children's relationships and observations without pushing them to express things they don't want to or talking about their families in ways that may create internal stress. Working with parents and caregivers is essential as these are nearly always children's source of safety.

Safety in all interactions with children can be promoted through consistency, trust, use of comfort items, narrating processes even to children who are very young, and validating emotions. In addition, paying attention to non-verbal cues and offering reassurance. It is important to introduce yourself to children to enhance trustworthiness and use age appropriate but truthful explanations. Seeking consent even from very small children models safety and trust. When things need to be done to children without consent, provide an explanation and offer apologies. It can be helpful to prepare children for what to expect through pictures or explanations and to listen carefully and respectfully to their fears and worries. It is commonplace to minimise or dismiss children's emotions, but to be trauma informed is to help them put words to these things and recognise them as valid and important. Children may also be able to contribute ideas on what may help them manage these fears and worries. Offer choice wherever possible, and when choices are limited, create some. Supporting children to integrate potentially traumatic events occurs through helping them gain a sense of agency and self-importance, as well as developing stories of themselves, their lives, and their emotions that they can comprehend (Box 12.3).

Box 12.3: Clinical example of trauma informed practice in a paediatric unit

Charlie is a nurse working on a paediatric unit. Charlie is providing care to Anthony who is 8. Anthony has experienced a series of intrusive medical procedures for an enduring condition and is increasingly distressed when admitted to the hospital because last time he found the pain unbearable. He has been admitted for another procedure, and his mum reports he has been having nightmares and wetting the bed.

In planning Anthony's care, Charlie focuses on a few things. Charlie finds it overwhelming when Anthony gets upset, and he often feels himself starting to panic. Charlie focuses on his breathing and reminds himself to stay focused on Anthony. Charlie takes care to ensure he remains calm and speaks in a gentle, soothing voice with Anthony. His calm demeanour seems to help Anthony feel more secure.

Charlie acknowledges Anthony's distress and fear. He doesn't dismiss it or minimise it or make promises. Instead, he listens and validates it and tries to focus on how they can make a plan together to get through the procedure. Charlie asks Anthony what will help and together they come up with a few strategies. Charlie wants to coach Anthony to take slow, deep breaths as this has been what has been helping him when he feels overwhelmed, but he knows this can be a lot for a child to comprehend. Instead, Charlie says, 'let's imagine you are blowing up a balloon. Can you blow it up long and slow and puff out your cheeks?' Charlie models the breathing exercise, doing it with Anthony.

When Charlie has built up some trust with Anthony, he tries to help him relax his body and become conscious of the sensations within it. He tries to do this by asking Anthony to pretend he is a bit of uncooked spaghetti – to make his body straight and stiff and to hold this tension. And then to relax like a piece of cooked spaghetti – making his whole body loose and floppy.

As part of their plan, Charlie ensures Anthony has his favourite toy with him during the procedure to provide a sense of security. When Anthony gets embarrassed about having a teddy, Charlie smiles and tells Anthony about his own teddy he has at home. Charlie asks Anthony if he would like to hold his hand while the doctor talks to him about the procedure. Anthony says no, so Charlie lets Anthony know he will stand nearby in case Anthony changes his mind.

Charlie acknowledges Anthony's feelings without minimising them. He says things like 'It's ok to be scared'. When appropriate, like when they are waiting for transfer, Charlie engages Anthony in simple games like 'I Spy' to both distract him and draw his attention back to the present moment and his surroundings. Charlie offers to tell Anthony stories of other kids who have been sick and who have been in the hospital to shift his focus and make him feel less alone. Charlie makes up stories about kids who have survived brave things and tells them while he takes Anthony's vital signs and tidies up his bed each day. Charlie tells Anthony that one day other kids will hear the story of Anthony and what he survived. Anthony likes this idea and helps Charlie figure out how that story should go.

After periods of distress, Charlie tries to talk to Anthony about what happened and to try to brainstorm together ways to cope in the future. Charlie reassures Anthony that it's okay to feel scared sometimes. Together they try out different sensory items to see if any of them feel helpful. They decide to choose five things they can try next time Anthony feels upset. They allocate each idea to one of his fingers to help him remember them. These include the balloons, the spaghetti, squeezing the teddy, seeking comfort, or imagining a safe place he can go in his mind. Together they describe and imagine the details of the safe place.

Alongside these interactions with Anthony, Charlie supports Anthony's parents. He engages them in activities and conversations and stays with Anthony while they speak to the doctors and have a break. Charlie shows an interest in Anthony's sister, asking her about her interests and hobbies and making sure she also feels included and important.

Through these grounding, distraction, and narrative holding approaches, Charlie builds trust with Anthony, gives him opportunities to have choice and input into care, is sensitive to the way his past experiences may impact, and helps Anthony find meaning in the potentially traumatic medical experiences.

Trauma informed care with young people

Young people have rich and complex inner worlds and ways of making sense of things. Often adolescence and young adulthood are the times when they most start to reflect on experiences of adversity or start to articulate their own understandings of things that have happened in their lives. But at this stage of the lifespan, even more than any other, trust is crucial. Young people who have experienced trauma are likely highly attuned to adults' capacity to recognise or be present with emotion or distress.

Trauma researchers have identified distinct ways that trauma during childhood and young adulthood can impact development, particularly in fundamental aspects of self-regulation, interpersonal interactions, emotion, attention and cognition, behavioural self-control, and identity formation (Ford et al., 2022; Van Der Kolk et al., 2019). In clinical settings, young people who have experienced trauma may present in extremes; their identity either forms around embracing trauma or rejecting it. Young people who have experienced trauma are in a liminal space between developing and developed. This is a difficult time for any young person, but it is made infinitely more complex by experiences of fear, betrayal, or helplessness. To be trauma informed when working with young people is to recognise how impactful trauma can be at this stage of life on identity formation, independence, and hope for the future.

Many young people are experimenting with their own power and independence. When trauma is woven into this, young people may respond in polarised ways: they may give away all power and present as small and helpless, or alternatively, they may demand power in interactions by dominating the interaction or presenting a façade they want the world to see. Our role as nurses and midwives is not to engage in a power struggle with young people but to let them have experiences of safe power. To be positioned as a person who has experienced trauma may take away power from them unless they are given a choice in the process. It can be helpful to let them control interactions, within reason, and to be as non-reactive as possible to extremes.

Being a young person also brings out big emotions; big feelings in response to trauma in the present, or big feelings in response to events in the present that trigger trauma from the past. Consider a young person who presents in enormous distress and expresses suicidality after a brief relationship break-up. It may be that their relational trauma from parental separation as a child is activated and they are unconsciously re-experiencing emotions that they never properly expressed as a child. Indeed, many childhood traumas do not show their conscious impacts until adolescence and early adulthood. As nurses and midwives, our role is to hold their emotions without overwhelm and to help them find ways to start to hold them themselves. In doing so, we should be cautious of shutting down emotions, infantilising them, or expecting them to have the regulation capacity of adults. Our role is to let young people express themselves and find their own meaning in events.

Working with young people in trauma informed ways requires awareness of how young people may express distress through a range of behaviours, including difficulties with school, organisational skills, friendships, risk-taking, distraction, anxiety, or anger, as well as disrupted sleep, eating, or bodily functions. Being curious, non-judgemental, and non-reactive goes a long way. Adolescents will often test our responses through dropping crumbs of ideas into interactions, either verbally or non-verbally, to see how we react. I imagine myself picking up each crumb and holding it gently, not pretending it doesn't exist but also not overreacting to its presence. For example, they may say 'what would you know' or 'what do you care' to see how we react, or they may try to shock us with information or silence. Try to stay steady in yourself, be curious about their experience, offer them power, and narrate the process as you go. For example, you might say 'I'd like to know more about that, is there anything more about it you feel like you could tell me?' or 'I am wondering how you feel about silence; I'm kind of ok about it and happy to just sit here with you, but would you rather I kept chatting to fill the space?'

You can try to match your language to the young person but don't try to be someone you are not. For example, you may use the words they use or ask them what would be a good way to say something if you aren't sure. It is also not uncommon that young people will find it unbearable to be engaged with a nurse or midwife for too long in conversations about emotive topics and any attempt to disengage or distract should also be respected. Ruptures in rapport may be more frequent, and these should be tolerated and, where possible, repaired. In young adulthood, people start to make sense of trauma and tell stories of their lives that shape them. For young people who have experienced trauma, the presence of an adult who shows genuine interest in their inner world – even briefly – and can tolerate uncomfortable thoughts and experiences is immensely powerful. The story they tell now may evolve over time but your response to it is crucial (Box 12.4).

Box 12.4: Clinical example of trauma informed practice in a school health setting

Kat is a Registered Nurse working in a high school with adolescents. Her job includes helping young people who are sick or injured at school as well as delivering immunisations and preventative healthcare. A 14-year-old student, Jordan, has been presenting to the school clinic on numerous occasions over the last few months with headaches and Kat suspects Jordan may be experiencing stress. Kat knows from the school staff that Jordan has spent time in foster care and now lives with his grandmother. Up until now, Kat has given Jordan basic first aid and offered for him to rest awhile before returning to class. Today, Kat decides to try to ask a bit more about what is going on for him.

Kat asks Jordan's permission to undertake more of an assessment. Jordan shrugs and agrees. Kat ensures they are in a private, quiet space where people won't come in and out. She has a phone, and she may have to answer it, so she tells Jordan that in advance. Kat asks about Jordan's medical history, asking him about any significant injuries, illnesses, or experiences. Kat asks Jordan detailed questions about the headaches, including their frequency, duration, intensity, and what precipitates them. She takes his pain seriously. Kat also acknowledges Jordan's pain directly by saying, 'It must be horrible to keep having such bad headaches'. When Jordan says 'it sucks', Kat asks Jordan about when it 'sucks' the most. Kat listens attentively to Jordan's concerns without interrupting, showing genuine interest. Kat uses open-ended questions to encourage Jordan to share more about his life. 'Can you tell me about anything that's been particularly stressful or difficult for you lately?' She maintains a non-judgemental attitude and pays attention to her body language, facial expressions, and tone of voice. At one point, Jordan gets frustrated and says, 'This is dumb'. He starts walking around the room towards the door. Kat doesn't react or try to stop him. When he turns to look at her, she holds his eye contact and says gently, 'I'd be really keen for you to stay a bit longer to talk more about how things are for you if it feels possible'. Jordan shrugs and sits back down.

Kat identifies a few key things that seem important. Firstly, Jordan describes a change in behaviour; he mentions that his grades have dropped, and he hasn't been sleeping well. He can't identify any cause of his headaches but says he feels worried about them. In addition, Jordan seems reluctant to engage his family. Kat asks if she can contact Jordan's grandmother and he quickly declines stating he doesn't want to worry her. Kat acknowledges Jordan's concerns about involving his grandmother and reassures him about confidentiality. She asks Jordan if there are other trusted adults he feels comfortable talking to. Jordan declines. Kat has to figure out what she should do next. She feels a bit stuck. She considers a few options:

- She could tell Jordan she is worried about him *[trustworthiness]*.
- She could ask Jordan more specific questions about his life, including telling him that she is wondering if the headaches are linked to past or present stressors *[this may indicate to Jordan that she is open to hearing difficult things]*.
- She could keep an open mind to other possibilities. It may be that Jordan has a physical health condition, is being bullied at school and taking refuge in

the clinic, or any number of other stressors, rather than family trauma *[it is important not to assume that trauma is the main issue in people's lives]*.

- She could explore what feels useful to Jordan about coming to the clinic and make a plan with Jordan about when and how often he comes *[collaboration]*.
- She could let Jordan know directly that she is ok with hearing difficult things if there is anything he wants to talk about and encourage him to talk more when he feels like it *[trustworthiness]*.
- She could ask Jordan what he thinks might be helpful going forward *[empowerment]*
- She could try to refer Jordan to a trauma-specific counsellor or school counsellor *[being trauma informed does not require nurses to be trauma counsellors]*.

Working with families in trauma informed ways

Part of working with infants, children, and young people is working with families. Families can be crucial places for healing from trauma, as well as sources of help and support. Family support can be one key part of buffering the impacts of potentially traumatic events from leading to trauma. Families can also experience secondary and vicarious trauma or be the sources of trauma. The relationships between families and trauma can be complex and we might not fully understand or know what is going on. Trauma can impact how families interact with us as nurses and midwives or how available they are to support the person who is accessing care. Families are likely under stress whenever a member is sick or hurt or during a significant life transition and how they are responding may not be their usual way of being. Trying to understand this is crucial for promoting safety within the family unit.

It can be helpful to advocate for infants, children, or young people by ensuring their needs are considered and given voice in conversations, even if they are not present. We can do this by saying things like 'I wonder how that may be for … (child/young person)'. Excluding when you have concerns about child well-being, you should also be led by families and their ways of being. You may need to check what is ok to talk about and not talk about. Stay conscious of power in interactions, for example, where is the child positioned in the space, and where are you positioned? Stay curious and gentle. It can be helpful to ask what everyone is worried about and what they think their child or young person may be worried about. Similarly, children and young people may worry about their parents or families, and it is important to create space for them to share these worries without leaping to reassurance. Questions like 'who worries the most?' may start to draw out family dynamics.

How to juggle families can be a big challenge in nursing and midwifery. It is usually not our job to be family therapists or determine how trauma may be impacting. However, it is our role to recognise that most traumas are healed relationally and that families can be a place where this occurs. Trauma also impacts whole families and communities, so it is important to not treat our patients as stand-alone entities who are not impacted by or impacting others. For all of us, the people we love and care for and are cared for by are crucial to all of our experiences, including recovery. As nurses and midwives, we always need to ask people about who they consider family and apply the same principles of trauma informed practice to all family and carers.

Trauma informed care of adults and older adults across settings

Trauma can impact adults in any setting. It is relevant to all healthcare. This is perhaps the most crucial point. Being TIC is relevant to all settings, regardless of why people are accessing care, and what their level of health or consciousness is.

I got an immunisation recently and the nurse administering it was busy. She was busy chatting to another practitioner about another patient, preparing the immunisation while their conversation continued, and hardly looking at me. I was watching how she prepared the immunisation, feeling nervous about her lack of attentiveness as well as uncomfortable about the conversation about another patient. When she had prepared the immunisation, she came over, pushed up my sleeve, and inserted it into my upper arm without skipping a beat in her conversation. I was shocked. The immunisation didn't hurt, and I am sure her preparation was adequate, but the lack of human contact was deeply unsettling. I didn't feel traumatised by the encounter; nothing bad had happened to me. But I felt concerned that nursing work could occur in a way that invisibilised the patient to that extent. I also felt concerned that I hadn't said anything. I hadn't said anything because of power. Because she held the power in that moment and I felt compliant. And because I feared that if I caused any trouble, it could be me that they were chatting about later in front of other patients. As nurses and midwives, our work-world can feel familiar and comfortable. This can lead us to forget how strange it can feel for patients to enter this world. To be trauma informed is to look in on our care as outsiders and to imagine how it might feel to people. Alongside this, applying the principles in practice regardless of setting is crucial to ensuring people have positive experiences of care.

Sometimes people assume that by stages of adulthood, they will have their lives sorted and trauma under control. It can be confronting for adults to be in positions of vulnerability or to find experiences from the past reactivated during the dynamics of healthcare. Being trauma informed requires us to hold a sense of the whole person, who they were prior, what they are experiencing currently, and what they hope for their future. We care for people at moments in their lives where their defences can be either down or very activated due to whatever it is that brings them to care. Across the lifespan, our role remains one of regulation, acceptance, and noticing.

Much of the research on trauma is from working age adults, and increasingly young people. This means that how trauma presents in older people is less well known. Older people may be dismissed as being a bit eccentric or getting dementia if they report changes in perception or memory associated with trauma. The losses that can come with age, including loss of autonomy, loss of loved ones, and social standing, can exacerbate trauma, as well as reduce coping strategies. Many younger people exercise a lot or work a lot to escape trauma, but this can be less possible in older age. The effects of coping mechanisms such as alcohol or drug use, isolation, overeating, over-exercise, or stress as a response to trauma can also amplify physical health complaints in older adulthood. Older age can also alter the meaning that people attach to events and experiences. There is a transition of self that occurs in later years as social roles change which can be altered by trauma that occurred during early development of self.

Trauma in older age can be expressed in the same ways as at any stage of life but also through increased intrusive thoughts, memories, bad dreams, or preoccupation with death and suffering. Trauma may also present through physical pain or ailments. As nurses, we may be providing care to older people who have one of three experiences of trauma:

1 People may have experienced trauma earlier in their lives and have existing coping mechanisms, but aging may make these strategies less accessible or effective, or trauma-related symptoms may be exacerbated through medical illness, reduced physical ability, dependence, and fewer distractions.
2 People may have managed to never process earlier trauma but are blindsided by its effects in older age.
3 People may experience trauma later in life, including in care.

Many people live long periods of their lives without painful recollections of trauma, only to have them re-emerge later in life. Through normal processes of ageing (or through the vulnerability of care environments), effects of trauma can surface after decades of effective coping. Changes in memory associated with ageing can interrupt cognitive strategies or defence mechanisms that people have used throughout their earlier lives to reduce the impact of traumatic memories. Some of the incredible ways that the brain survives, such as shutting off memories from accessibility or hiding memories to make them less problematic, can be disrupted by ageing. In the same way that other parts of the body can lose their strength or soften, so it seems can the mechanisms that lock away memories. This means people may experience flashbacks or nightmares of things they haven't thought about or remembered previously. These can be intense, vivid, sensory experiences. The possible neuroscience behind these changes includes that the nerve cells that control memory, thinking, and judgement are altered during aging processes and there can be a decrease in the cortical area impacting rationalising trauma-related responses. The memory loss of dementia and conditions like Alzheimer's can mean that the past is more available than the recent. The accessibility of memories can also change so that short-term and recent storage can be impacted before longer-term areas. This can be problematic if trauma memories have been stored away for a lifetime as people can live past trauma as though it is happening now in the present.

Older people can also experience significant trauma in healthcare due to reliance upon care, loss of dignity, ageism, challenges to interpersonal safety due to loss of senses, the need for physical care, a decrease in trust in their own body or mind, themes of interactions which may centre on illness, loss and worry, and a loss of independence and control. The injury or illness itself may be more likely to be traumatic because of what is at stake in relation to the future and ongoing independence or functioning. Awareness of these dynamics is crucial for trauma informed nursing care. Patience and respect are also incredibly important; older people may be sensitive to being dismissed or patronised by younger professionals (Box 12.5).

Box 12.5: Clinical example of loss of personhood in older age

Dotty is in her 90s and fit as can be. She had a fall at the hairdresser and broke her hip and was admitted to hospital for a lengthy stay. Her mood dropped very low during her admission, and she feels like 'just another 90-year-old with a broken hip who may never recover'. Previously, she was living a full life; she plays cards, goes to book club, has friends, is interested in world events, and is fit and healthy. She begins to worry she may die in the hospital because she feels invisible. The overwhelming sense of helplessness, fear, and loss of power Dotty experiences is akin to a potentially traumatic event. She describes that the nurses are nice to her, she isn't mistreated, but she doesn't feel seen or known. She begins to feel like a small child again and over time starts to hope that she dies. She is experiencing trauma associated with a loss of personhood.

Nurses and midwives have a role in recognising who people are and what might be happening for them based on their experiences in the past. It is important to know an older person's story enough to enable adjustments in care and to recognise the symbolic nature of things that may have been built over a lifetime (Craftman et al., 2020). For example, older people who may have not had enough food during periods of war and develop dementia may try to carry food items with them or hide food in their rooms. Or a person who escaped violence as a young person may sleep with their shoes on in case they need to escape in a hurry. They may speak of losses from long ago as though they are current or mistake us for people from their past. Being able to hold these experiences in the context of what might have happened for someone is just as important as knowing why they occur. Older people may have lived through multiple losses or potentially traumatic events that can be reactivated in care, and they may also be very worried about their future. Recognising the wholeness of older people and their experiences is part of being trauma informed.

References

Craftman, Å. G., Swall, A., Båkman, K., Grundberg, Å., & Hagelin, C. L. (2020). Caring for older people with dementia reliving past trauma. *Nursing Ethics, 27*(2), 621–633. https://doi.org/10.1177/0969733019864152

D'Agata, A. L., Young, E. E., Cong, X., Grasso, D. J., & McGrath, J. M. (2016). Infant medical trauma in the neonatal intensive care unit (IMTN): A proposed concept for science and practice. *Advances in Neonatal Care, 16*(4), 289–297. https://doi.org/10.1097/ANC.0000000000000309

Ford, J. D., Charak, R., Karatzias, T., Shevlin, M., & Spinazzola, J. (2022). Can developmental trauma disorder be distinguished from posttraumatic stress disorder? A symptom-level person-centred empirical approach. *European Journal of Psychotraumatology, 13*(2), 2133488. https://doi.org/10.1080/20008066.2022.2133488

Lyons-Ruth, K., Dutra, L., Schuder, M. R., & Bianchi, I. (2006). From infant attachment disorganization to adult dissociation: Relational adaptations or traumatic experiences? *Psychiatric Clinics of North America, 29*(1), 63–86. https://doi.org/10.1016/j.psc.2005.10.011

Van Der Kolk, B., Ford, J. D., & Spinazzola, J. (2019). Comorbidity of developmental trauma disorder (DTD) and post-traumatic stress disorder: Findings from the DTD field trial. *European Journal of Psychotraumatology, 10*(1), 1562841. https://doi.org/10.1080/20008198.2018.1562841

13 Supporting after potentially traumatic events

Sometimes, or often, as nurses and midwives, we are looking after people who have recently experienced potentially traumatic events. This may include, as part of organised disaster responses, caring for people brought into hospital after traumatic accidents or experiences, people recovering from life-changing illnesses or procedures, or people whose lives have changed in any number of significant ways.

Our initial response should always focus on empathy and validation. This requires us to slow down and manage our own worries enough to be present and recognise the importance of acknowledging traumatic events, demonstrating sensitivity, and being led by the person. First, it can be helpful to validate ('this is a really hard thing to be going through' or 'you have been through a lot'). Be curious but not investigative, for example, you might say 'what do you think it is important for me to know?' or 'would it be helpful to talk more about it?' Only after we have demonstrated care and listening should we move to any reassurance or planning. Responding to trauma in the moment requires skills of kindness and sensitivity. It requires us to go slower in our selves than usual healthcare interactions or social interactions, where distressing events may be glossed over or reassurance offered. When we witness or hear about trauma, we need to hold the moment with care and give it due space and recognition.

Responding in the aftermath of trauma might mean offering support or advocating for services. It might mean referring to or encouraging the person to seek help. Or it may mean working on a care plan that addresses their needs in your service, in your care, and going forward. It may mean fostering hope and a sense that the world is predictable and safe. It is usual to feel distressed after a potentially traumatic event of any kind. People may feel teary or agitated. They may be unable to sleep. They may have memories of it playing over and over in their minds. Depending on what the event was, they may feel guilt or anger or shame or regret or any other strong negative emotion. They may feel overwhelmed by the way they feel, distressed by the replaying in their minds, and have a sense that things will never be ok again. They are trapped in the moment of trauma and not yet able to imagine a future beyond it. Kindness, connection, and understanding are helpful to anyone in this state. As nurses and midwives, we have an opportunity to help people understand their experience and make it feel more manageable, but only once they are ready. Table 13.1 presents an acronym to support responses. The steps may seem basic, but they can be helpful to have something to anchor our minds in the moment when we need to respond to someone's distress. Responding requires us to slow down and ensure we are supporting people in the ways they need.

DOI: 10.4324/9781003530770-16

Table 13.1 ALIVE acronym for responding after trauma

A	**Accept and acknowledge**	Accepting and acknowledging requires us to accept whatever the person is feeling or thinking so that they can also accept it. It might look something like 'You have been through something really confronting, what you are feeling is absolutely ok'
L	**Listen**	Listening is always important. In this context, it is about listening to what the person tells us they want and need, but it also involves listening to how they talk about experiences and what they emphasise. Through really listening, we can get a sense of what parts of the events or experience are causing them the most distress, we can also get clues about the ways they are talking to themselves about trauma, and we can start to identify what kind of support they may need. Listening can require us to sit with things they tell us that are uncomfortable, including their own sense of guilt or blame. It is important not to jump to reframing or reassuring without first listening in detail
I	**Inquire**	It is important to ask and not assume. Once you have listened and got a bit of a sense of things, it is helpful to ask questions. You can ask general questions, or you can ask specific questions about what you have noticed. For example, you might say 'what is the bit that is distressing you the most?" or you might say "it seems that there is something about that particular moment that keeps going around in your mind?' Inquiring is about opening up space for them to continue to share with you. They may feel overwhelmed by what they feel and assume you will be too. Inquiring gives the message that we can handle what they are thinking and feeling, and we are willing to hold it
V	**Validate**	Validation is similar to acceptance but it provides more of an empathic reassurance that you understand what someone is trying to tell you and that it makes sense to you. After traumatic events, people may feel that what they are worried about or feeling is silly or too much or doesn't make sense. Validation is crucial for connection. You might say something like 'I can hear that you think you shouldn't have responded that way, but I want to reassure you that it makes sense to me that you did'. However, you don't have to agree with the person's interpretation to validate; for example, if someone is blaming themselves, you might say, 'It is common for people to blame themselves after big things happen. I know you feel that way, but I want you to know that I do not think that was your fault'
E	**Explain**	Explaining is where knowledge of trauma comes in the most, but it is also the stage we need to be most careful with. People can feel really lost in their responses to traumatic events. Sometimes they feel nothing, or they feel too much, and either way they often feel blindsided by the experiences and their response. Explaining can be a way of throwing them a lifeboat in the midst of overwhelm by letting them know that how they feel now will settle and that you have seen people survive such things before. It may be helpful to initially talk about trauma in more detached ways so that you can identify whether a framework of trauma aligns with people's worldview. For example, 'Things that are life-changing, like trauma, can feel initially overwhelming before the initial waves start to settle'. Referring to other people's responses to trauma and how trauma memories impact them may be helpful. For example, 'Often people play the events over and over in their minds while their brain tries to make sense of them. This is difficult, but it's also part of how we cope'

Debriefing trauma in healthcare

Sometimes trauma occurs within healthcare, and the role of nurses or midwives is to help people make sense of what happened. This can be relevant to acute care settings like emergency or intensive care but can also relate to any part of care. A less obvious example is birth. Many experiences of giving birth are potentially traumatic. That doesn't mean they end up resulting in trauma, but as events they often overwhelm people's sense that they can cope and can shatter ideas of what they expected or wanted. Birth can be a contradictory experience for people, both incredible and joyful, while also potentially traumatic.

Nearly all people who give birth value opportunities to talk about the birth process with health professionals (usually midwives). In the places I have worked and birthed, it hasn't historically been usual practice to offer birth debriefs, although I know this is shifting in many places. Traditionally, a midwife or doctor may come and see you afterwards and have a sweeping general conversation about what happened, but this is different from an intentional and collaborative sense-making. This is despite the fact that such events can be most active in our minds and memories in the first week or two after exposure; sleep can also feel impossible during these same weeks; and the link between difficult birth experiences (including disappointment or unexpected levels of pain or intervention) and postnatal mental health. Debriefing after an event like birth serves a very different purpose from a medical debrief that occurs to ensure safe practice and understanding of decision-making processes.

When, as a nurse, I saw parents on the postnatal ward in the days after birth, they nearly always just wanted to talk about the birth over and over. Their faces would look at me in ways that appeared activated when I asked about birth, curious if I was safe to tell the whole story to, looking for cues that I was interested and not going to offer reassurance or dismissal. Talking about the details of events is a way to make sense of what has happened, make the incomprehensible comprehensible, and develop a shared narrative. It should happen when people feel ready. As a couple, a family, or an individual, they were forming a shared story of the birth. These conversations are of critical importance for reducing ongoing trauma, regardless of the objective events.

I would offer people the chance to talk through the birth, making space for any feelings of disappointment or anger or surprise, alongside feelings of awe and joy, supporting a sense of linearity in the story and identifying any questions they wanted answers for. If they had emerging narratives that were negative about themselves (e.g. 'I should have waited longer before asking for pain relief' or 'I don't understand why I let that happen' or 'I feel embarrassed by how loud I was'), then I would offer generous alternatives and watch whether they were able to consider a different perspective (e.g. 'you probably made a decision that letting that happen was the best way to get through?' or 'The hormones of birth sometimes amplify emotions in preparation of bonding with the baby, do you think it could have been that?' and so on). I would tell parents that telling the story to each other was important in trying to make sense of the memories and that this will settle. It takes about a week for the intensity of 're-living' the moment to settle, it won't stay as it is right now, and it is important to check in after that about what parts are still lingering.

Like any other trauma, it is about the experience and effect, not the event. Births which may be traumatic may not always appear so to others. They may include feelings of powerlessness or fear or betrayal of body, of self, and of others. People may also experience fight, flight, or freeze responses that they later feel shame about, for example, becoming angry at staff or support people, trying to get away or deciding they 'can't do this', or becoming passive and not advocating for themselves and their wishes. In line with knowledge of trauma, when we can't fight, we have to activate other defence mechanisms. We might turn to those around us to protect us (in the case of birth that might be midwives, doctors, or a partner), but if we feel betrayed by them (because they don't seem to help us or listen) and also dependent upon them (because we feel stuck, scared, or overwhelmed), then we can feel alone and freeze – activating a dissociative response. I've worked with many parents for whom this was what lingered – a sense that they should have done something to advocate for themselves or their partner. But they didn't. I would suggest to people that they couldn't have done something; their brain was saving them in the best way it knew how, by removing them from the present, and when this happens, actions are limited. Understanding why you didn't do anything differently is crucial as it interrupts loops that can form in the brain about self-blame or confusion.

I think of this process during debriefing as palpating for stuckness, gently palpating the memory to see which bit is causing a problem. The idea is a gentle pushing, without causing pain, noticing which bits people react to. As trusted clinicians whom people share their experiences, there are some intentional things we can do in conversation to try to help with 'stuck' bits of memories. Stuck bits are usually parts that we can't make sense of, so we just keep going over and over them. Usually, they present themselves when people are talking; people keep looping back to this moment, or the story seems to take a sudden turn at that moment. Or they are talking and then suddenly they are crying. These are clues that you have palpated a stuck bit. You can also ask directly – *are there bits you keep replaying?* Like a knot in a muscle that causes pain or restricts our movement, sometimes rubbing the muscle is enough to smooth out the knot and help it blend back into the overall muscle. We want to relationally help smooth out the 'knot' in the memory and to do that we can listen to the stuck bit, notice it, and explore the thoughts and emotions that stem from it. We can help the person find meaning in it and try to gently link it to the other bits of the story or widen the person's perception of that moment a tiny bit to allow some more possibilities in. While these approaches may seem natural in conversation, in practice they can differ a lot from usual responses. When people tell us something distressing that happened, the 'usual' response is to get the sweeping overview and try to reassure them, skip over the distressing details, or give them opposing perspectives. This (while appropriate in some circumstances) doesn't always help potentially traumatic memories settle and can be experienced as invalidating.

Box 13.1 includes a few examples of bits of birth stories that appeared 'stuck' upon debrief. The same ideas apply to moments of potentially traumatic memories in other contexts too. Nurses in all kinds of settings will be hearing recent experiences people have had of feeling sick or hurt, or trying to access care, or having surgery, or being in the hospital, and there can be moments of 'stuckness' in all of these memories, giving us opportunities to be purposefully trauma informed in our responses.

Box 13.1: Clinical examples of 'stuck' trauma memories

Annie's baby was born via a forceps delivery after a long labour. By the time the baby was assisted out, Annie was exhausted. Annie is telling the story of the moment her baby was born and how the forceps fell to the floor. She says that in that moment, she thought her baby's head had fallen off with the forceps. Annie becomes distressed in this part of the story. Her eyes glaze, and she cries and looks away, and the story fizzles out. She is stuck in that moment. Her baby's head had not fallen off and she knows this because she was holding the wriggling and happy baby while she told the story, but it doesn't matter what the facts were. In her mind, that moment just plays over and over.

Heidi had a normal vaginal delivery in a midwifery-run birth centre. The birth went as she had hoped, but she started to bleed after the delivery. She is telling this part of the story when she becomes upset. 'I looked down and blood was every-where', she says. Her husband is next to her as she tells the story, and he reaches for her hand. I get the feeling he has heard this story many times before and he knows this is the upsetting bit. Heidi accepts his hand, but it doesn't seem to soothe her; she is looking at me intently and speaking rapidly. She tells me that no one was helping her. 'But I was right there', says her husband quietly. It is like she doesn't hear him. In her memory, she was all alone and bleeding. This is where she is stuck.

Kirrily had a vaginal birth. She tells the story pretty matter-of-factly and without too many signs of distress. She experienced some significant tearing and required an epidural to repair her perineum. She was awake throughout the repair. She describes her legs in stirrups and doctors gathered around. 'They brought the students in!' she exclaims, 'I can still see their faces. It must have been so terrible as they looked really shocked'. Her whole face changes and her eyes drift off. This is where she is stuck.

Debriefing is like a zipper. We try to zip the zipper and notice how it slides. It can sometimes feel difficult to start and we need to line the bits up to bring them together. Sometimes, once it is zipping, it hits a bump and can't keep going. We go back and forth, trying to smooth the lump and line up the teeth so the zip can smoothly slide on.

To start debriefing conversations in the context of birth, but equally applicable to any context, I might ask people to tell me the story. Often this can feel over-whelming, and they may say, 'I don't know where to start', to which I respond, 'start wherever you feel like and we can work out the rest'. We can support them to find a beginning or to begin from wherever they start and work backwards or forwards to start to develop some linearity in things that feel disparate and scattered. Or if I want to be more targeted, I might say things like 'which bits do you keep reliving?' And then I try to stay with that moment rather than rushing ahead in the story. I might say directly, 'can we stay with that moment for a bit?' and ask more detailed questions like 'What do you remember about what others did?' or 'What do you remember about what you did?' or 'What do you remember was happening around you at that moment?' or 'What decisions do you remember making?' or 'What happened imme-diately before/after that?' Sometimes it is like taking a photograph of the moment of stuckness, zooming in on the stuckness, and then zooming out to understand the context together to try to understand it.

As they talk, I listen and I notice. I notice how they sit, when they cry, and what words they use. I try to hold the threads of the story to support cohesion. I try to restore some sense of safety or trust in themselves and others by suggesting alternative perspectives of what *may* have been occurring or why. I find reassurance is not helpful in this situation; at best, it seems to have no impact upon people and at worst, feels invalidating. Try to validate emotions and thoughts – notice when people mention them and repeat them. Notice moments of resistance – times when they tried to assert control or change the course of events. And consider any aspects of fear or distress or betrayal. Don't give the sense that the story is messy or unmanageable. It is important that we reinforce the cohesion and tolerability of hearing it. In identifying the stuck moments and gently exploring the thoughts and feelings that surround them, we can start to support their integration into the wider story of what happened. When they fit in the narrative, they will no longer be stuck.

Understanding how traumatic memories work is important in trying to help people wrestle with them. Ruminating is a way for the brain to regain control and make sense of an experience. Our brains want to avoid traumatic things happening again and figure out what they can do differently. This is a usual process, but it isn't rational. The memory swirls around and around until it makes sense. We want traumatic memories to be integrated into narratives we hold of our lives and our pasts, not encapsulated as a horrific moment that we replay that doesn't make sense in the narrative or leads to flashbacks and intrusive reliving. To achieve this, we need to help people link the potentially traumatic bit to other bits of the story in ways that make sense. This is not about seeking out the facts of what happened (although sometimes this can really help people), but about finding a narrative that is acceptable of what *might have* happened. This means that when we identify a stuck bit, we can try to stay with that bit of the story a bit more, lean into it a bit to understand the threads, and then gently see how it can link back into the whole narrative. These might sound like in-depth trauma interventions because I am breaking them down to their moment-to-moment pieces, but they are actually just intentional conversations that can be woven into existing practice.

Throughout any debriefing, it is important to support grounding. This refers to helping the person return to the present and to leave the unsafe space of the past. What works to help people feel grounded differs for everyone, but some suggestions include getting people to blink and feel their eyelashes move, to notice where their hands are, and to squeeze them. Sometimes people like to hold something and turn it around in their hand or to push their feet onto the ground and wriggle their toes. Breathing strategies can help. But essentially anything that helps you return to your body, consciousness, and present. When debriefing with children or young people, providing some sort of fiddle activity or sensory item can help support them to find ways to ground themselves.

The following scenario gives an example of starting a debrief process, breaking down each comment to link to the intentionality. It is not a perfect example (no debrief or conversation ever is), but I've included it here to normalise the approach and highlight the ways it may differ from a usual interaction.

Debriefing birth experience

In this scenario, a midwife (Effie) is having a debrief with her patient (Alex), a week after birth. You may imagine this is one of their postpartum visits as part of a continuity of care model. The transcript is long, so I have just included two short snippets here with some analysis of the intent behind what Alex shares and how Effie responds added in bold.

Midwife (Effie):	*Your body is healing really well, I am wondering how you have been feeling about the birth?* **(introduces the topic and identifies the importance of talking about the birth)**
Parent (Alex):	*I can't believe it's been a week already. In some ways it's been the longest week of my life but in others it feels like time has stopped and I'm still there.* **(some stuckness is already apparent in the warping of time)**
Effie:	*Still in the hospital?* **(staying with the details to pace the story)**
Alex:	*Yes, still in that room. The one … I don't even know where it was! I can't remember getting there!* **(lack of coherence)**
Effie:	*So many things happened …* **(taking a guess at what Alex may be trying to say)**
Alex:	*It feels like a dream. It just keeps playing in my mind.*
Effie:	*It is not uncommon for women to say that they just keep reliving the birth over and over.* **(normalising and building safety).**
Alex:	*I know I am driving Jim mad because I keep asking him questions about what happened.*
Effie:	*It's really important to just keep telling the story until it starts to make sense. It helps the brain store the memory in different way.* **(normalising ideas of trauma and memories)**
Alex:	*I just … I just … I felt so scared*
Effie:	*I can imagine you felt scared.* **(validating).** *I wonder if it might be helpful to go through it together? Start at the beginning and try and piece it together?* **(purposeful and pacing)**
Alex:	*I remember I was so excited… I remember ringing delivery ward when I was first in labour.* **(launches straight in, indicating the memory is still close to the surface)**
Effie:	*What did you feel in your body that made you know it was labour? What was the first thing?* **(slowing down the story and focusing in on the experience not the events)**
Effie:	*Did you feel scared?* **(testing out an emotion)**
Alex:	*No. I wasn't scared. Kind of more annoyed maybe like no one understood what was happening.*
Effie:	*What about Jim? What was he doing at this bit?* **(widening awareness to surrounds and who else was there, as trauma can give tunnel vision)**
Alex:	*He was there, he was with me. Maybe he had to move the car but then he was with me, just reassuring and rubbing my back. Yeah, he was there.*
Effie:	*So, Jim was with you, and you were sitting in the foyer, feeling things weren't going how they were meant to.* **(creating an image of the moment so they can study it together).** *Were other people around? How long did that bit go for?*
Alex:	*There were people around, I think. I remember people walking past. I have no idea how long we were there. The pain got worse and started*

	to feel overwhelming and so we went back into the ward. **(moving on from that moment with reduced stuckness)**
Effie:	*Were you in a room?* **(attempting to orient)**
Alex:	*Yeah, we were in a room. Even though the pain was worse we felt a bit more back on track. At least I did. Jim hadn't eaten anything, so my mum brought him some food and then she kind of just stayed … so she was there too.*
Effie:	*Were you happy to have her there?* **(palpating for emotion)**
Alex:	*It wasn't the plan, but I didn't mind. I kind of just went into my own world you know, focusing on my body and the breathing. I had one of those big ball things and was sitting on that for … I don't know, maybe hours (laughs)*
Effie:	*You just really went into your own body and focused on what you needed to do … it's amazing.* **(focusing on strengths and acts of resistance)**

When I read through the full transcript of this birth debrief with midwives in a trauma informed debriefing workshop, many were surprised that I had chosen this scenario as an example. In the story, Alex has a long but straightforward birth which ends without incident. They talked about how to them it sounded like a 'textbook' birth, not a traumatic birth. But this is why I chose this example. It reminds us that how people experience the events is more important than the events themselves. We can get distracted by the events and their details and miss how it feels moment to moment. Being able to listen to the minutiae of experiences and tease out the emotion is crucial for being sensitive to trauma. While usually in nursing and midwifery we may be debriefing objectively more distressing events than Alex's birth, we can't assume what is traumatic to people.

The midwife in this example was very intentional with her responses and what parts of the story she picked up on. She focused on holding the thread of the story and identifying emotions and experiences that were apparent within the events. The purpose of this is targeted; it aids the fostering of a cohesive and comprehensible story, so it is not stored long-term as a traumatic memory. These same principles apply to any potentially traumatic event – there is benefit in holding the story with someone and trying to piece together all the bits, identifying emotions and bits that feel incomprehensible. The intent is not for you to explain or fix these bits but to move them into conscious awareness so that people can make their own sense of them.

Responding to trauma that occurs outside of healthcare contexts

Nurses, and sometimes midwives, may be responding to people who have experienced trauma from events outside of the healthcare context. This is often the case in settings like emergency departments, but it can also occur within communities in response to disaster events. Disasters occur quickly, usually without warning, and cause destruction or a serious threat. They can be naturally occurring (for example, earthquakes, storms, floods, or fires) or man-made events (like chemical explosions, train derailments, or plane crashes). Disasters usually cause losses for whole communities or groups and may exceed the capacity to cope or respond. Nurses are often involved in preparing for and responding to disasters.

The principles of responding in these contexts are the same as those in healthcare. In the period after a potentially traumatic event, acute stress reactions or distress are to be expected. Most people benefit from support, reassurance, and resources. The initial priority is practical support and provision of resources (food, shelter, money, communication). People may also require emotional reassurance, space to process events through retelling the story, or they may not want to talk at all. While we may think of trauma after disasters, we shouldn't assume that this will be people's experience. Fostering a sense of hope and self and collective efficacy is required, alongside respecting people's belief systems and engagement with the community. This can occur through helping people identify what they need to do with a focus on short-term goals and needs, supporting community engagement, and listening to community ways of being, while also encouraging self-care. It can be hard to think very far in the future at all when assumptions of safety are shattered, so we may be helping people survive in momentary increments, figuring out what they need right now and in the next few minutes, and then hours, and then days.

It is 'normal' to feel traumatised after being exposed to a potentially traumatic event. It doesn't mean the person will have residual trauma. Many people and communities will never think of their experiences as trauma. One of the key roles nurses and midwives can offer, beyond immediate healthcare, is to support people while this initial response settles. Being trauma informed doesn't require us to push people to talk about experiences or overly pathologise distress. It requires us to recognise the powerlessness and helplessness of potentially traumatic events and to try to restore a sense of power and hope, relationally. This should always be led by the person's priorities, supporting coherence and self-care, along with validating, listening, and recognising resistance.

Responses to disasters are embedded in culture and community. People from rural areas may be impacted differently or conceptualise needs differently than people from urban areas, people may identify their experiences individually or collectively, and communities may have experienced cumulatively hardships that alter how they respond to the current disaster. Our role should always be to be humble, available, and not assume how events will impact individuals or groups.

14 Vicarious trauma and radicalising self-care

Traditionally, health professionals have been expected to be 'detached' from our work, to avoid being unable to cope. Trauma informed care (TIC) undoes this assumption by encouraging awareness, empathy, and therapeutic presence. Therefore, there is a need to ensure other strategies are in place to help us manage the demands of our roles.

When understanding trauma, it is important to acknowledge the ways trauma can also impact staff. Many people who work in healthcare have experienced trauma in their own lives. We may be 'triggered' during our work or vulnerable to retraumatisation at work. We may also experience trauma through witnessing events, pain, and loss, or from participating in the delivery of interventions, treatments, or care. Some things that happen at work are traumatic. We may witness a baby die during birth or a procedure go wrong. A patient or staff member may attack us or we may see horrific injuries. We may be forced to do things that feel immoral like hold someone down and administer an injection or force a child to take a medication. These experiences can feel traumatic and may lead to traumatic effects. We also carry responsibilities for the lives of others which at times can be difficult to make sense of. For example, nurses found responsible for adverse events or clinical errors often live with fear, shame, guilt, anxiety, insomnia, or hypervigilance (Hall & Scott, 2012). Despite how tough many nurses and midwives may feel, we are not immune to the things we see. For example, in one study, up to 48% of nurses in intensive care units were identified to experience symptoms of PTSD (Sanchez et al., 2019).

TIC is about more than just how we treat people who access care. It is a way of thinking about workplaces, workforces, and organisations. Once someone views things through a trauma informed lens, it doesn't make sense to not also do so with colleagues, self, and staff. The well-being of nurses and midwives is therefore a critical component of delivering effective TIC. Even when we are resilient, we are also impacted by our work.

Healthcare workers in general have higher rates of lifetime trauma than the general population, increasing the risk of retraumatisation. Not everyone will bring existing and historic trauma to the work, but many do. Nurses are known to report high rates of abuse in childhood and adulthood, particularly emotional abuse. Nurses report higher rates of childhood emotional abuse (Choi et al., 2022) and sexual and physical abuse (Saunders & Adams, 2014) than the general population. Histories of trauma do not equate to weakness in the workforce, and they may contribute to empathy, care, and trauma sensitivity. However, such experiences may also predispose workers to secondary or vicarious trauma (VT) occurring in the course of their work. There are various terms used to describe indirect ways trauma can impact nurses and midwives. For example, secondary trauma can occur from hearing about things we don't directly

DOI: 10.4324/9781003530770-17

experience. We often experience this from the stories we hear and share about things that happen. We can experience this from handovers, hearing people's stories, or witnessing the effects of trauma. We may also experience compassion fatigue. This refers to the loss of empathy and care that can develop over time, usually from emotional exhaustion or overwork. Compassion fatigue is a form of secondary trauma where repeatedly helping people who have experienced trauma can lead to fatigue and decreased capacity for empathy or care. Without adequate breaks or support, our brains become tired from constantly caring, and to protect us, they may shut down some of the automatic processes of empathy. Similarly, burnout can occur from a sense that our work becomes futile. Maybe because patients just keep streaming in the door or because our workplace doesn't acknowledge or support us enough. Burnout refers to a syndrome characterized by emotional exhaustion, depersonalization, and reduced feelings of personal accomplishment. It results from sustained exposure or work with populations which are vulnerable or suffering, without adequate structural support. Perhaps we start to feel like our work is pointless or that no matter what we do, it will make no difference. Burnout is characterised by a loss of interest in our work or personal life, feeling like we are just going through the motions. Both burnout and compassion fatigue can result in a loss of motivation for work or avoidance of patient care or engagement, as well as having implications for our physical and mental health. We can usually notice the change in ourselves, and even if we feel helpless to alter it, we can usually appropriately locate that the 'issue' is a reaction to the work.

The systemic tensions nurses and midwives face in their work can also be a source of secondary trauma. These tensions can be amplified when we are attempting to be trauma informed within wider systems that aren't. It is painful to be labelled as traumatising for being part of a system, even if we actively try to practice differently.

In 2021 I wrote about the challenges of being trauma informed within systems or services that aren't (Isobel, 2021). It was a time when I felt very disheartened about 'the system' and I was wondering about the futility of striving to be trauma informed if the wider context of services wasn't. I was witnessing a form of gaslighting, where services had up posters stating things like 'This is a trauma informed service' and yet people were still feeling dehumanised or disempowered within care, replicating and creating trauma dynamics. I was also aware of a tension for clinicians. I felt like talking about TIC put an expectation on them to be humanistic and sensitive, when so much of what they were doing was trying to counteract the things that were out of their control.

Some days it felt like everyone walking into the hospital was slipping on a puddle on the floor from a tap that was left on, and I had been tasked with mopping the floor. While I was mopping, I was getting criticised for not mopping fast enough or well enough, getting blamed for people slipping on the puddle, trying to help people after they slipped, trying not to slip myself, and at the same time feeling incredibly frustrated that no one would just turn off the tap. In the worst moments, it felt as though those in power were watching the tap overflow, making no plan to turn it off. Instead, they told staff it was everyone's responsibility to mop – and if anyone slipped, it was our fault for not mopping well enough. It felt … futile. Perhaps this was burnout.

And then at the end of my long day mopping, I was soaked, exhausted, and expected to return tomorrow to mop some more. I started to feel tired of hearing about trauma and trying to help. Perhaps this was compassion fatigue.

But it wasn't futile. It is important that we acknowledge the 'taps that are left running' in our services, which are commonly the ways services are funded, staffed, and set up. Sometimes our 'taps' also include the limitations of medical systems and treatments or other pressures on services. It is important to acknowledge how hard and tiring it is to work in such systems and the moral injuries it can cause, alongside providing staff with adequate training, breaks, supervision, and workforce opportunities. The exhaustion I felt was from trying to mop the floor, look after the folks who had slipped, AND turn off the tap. This is not something wrong with me; this is just too much work. This is why implementation requires buy-in, plans, a gang of implementors, and levels of targeted action. I don't want to take this puddle metaphor too far, but the other thing is that the puddle from the taps left running is a distraction from what people are there for. People come to hospitals or healthcare settings because they need help or to improve or maintain their health; ideally, they don't get harmed in the process. I don't think it is futile to provide care in ways that acknowledge the puddle, try to reduce it causing harm to people, and help them if they do slip in it, all while continuing to advocate that the taps get turned off. The futile feeling came from exhaustion, and it is important to acknowledge that it is tiring and that the responsibility doesn't lie solely on staff. People working within services, including nurses and midwives, are often faced with an unspoken choice to concede to the dominant paradigms of the systems we work within or to actively disrupt them. It is not possible to fully prevent retraumatisation within systems of care without wider political and social change. But at the same time, engaging with a nurse or midwife who is trauma informed and trauma sensitive makes a huge difference to how people experience care. Thus, we can do what we can, and we can look after people accessing care, ourselves and each other, even if we aren't the source of the water (Box 14.1).

Box 14.1: Covid-19 and nursing trauma

During the global pandemic of Covid-19 in 2020/2021, nurses were positioned as heroes. People lined their balconies and clapped and cheered; there was widespread gratitude and admiration. The graffiti artist Banksy even painted a mural. Nurses were briefly superheroes. It was an amazing time to be a nurse. In the hospital where I worked, we wore scrubs and protective equipment with pride. We were exhausted and scared but we were appreciated. At the university where I also worked, enrolments in nursing doubled. But there were problems with this image. If we paint nurses as selfless and giving heroes who live to care, we create a disconnect between the ideal and the reality. The reality is that these are hard jobs. That often nurses and midwives are working in short-staffed and under-resourced contexts providing care to people in all sorts of predicaments, who are not always happy to receive it.

Alongside the hero discourse, the pandemic also brought attention to the workplace trauma faced by nurses. The International Council of Nurses (ICN) declared a mass trauma event for the world's nurses due to exposure to deadly disease, nurse deaths, overstretched staff, psychological distress, and attacks by anti-vaccinators. The ICN suggested that Covid-19 was a 'unique and complex form of trauma' for the nursing profession and called for governments to act to protect nurses. The momentum of this global attention was an opportunity to raise awareness of the stress and trauma faced by nurses long before the pandemic.

Nurses and midwives have always faced dilemmas related to the ethical care of patients and their own safety. They have always borne witness to suffering and at times had to contribute to that suffering through invasive procedures.

Foli et al. (2020) argue that nurses have long suffered from what they term 'insufficient resource trauma'. This occurs from not having the staff, supplies, knowledge, or support to undertake our roles in ways that fulfil ethical or professional responsibilities. Inadequate staffing levels contribute to this unique form of workplace trauma. While many professions could claim this term and declare that they lack the resources to do their roles well, the aspect that makes this more potentially 'traumatic' for nurses and midwives is the close proximity to the vulnerability and need of patients. The choice between continuing or leaving can feel like a life-or-death one as nurses witness people suffering or dying in their care due to a perceived lack of care or support from governments. This forms a component of betrayal and stuckness, known to be inherent to complex trauma experiences. The trauma nurses and midwives face is therefore direct from what they witness, but also indirect, caused by what people don't see of their work and what they have to hold alongside the work. The pandemic highlighted these experiences, but it wasn't the source of them.

Vicarious trauma occurs beneath consciousness

Vicarious trauma (VT) is a unique way we can be impacted by work. As Rachel Remen observes: 'The expectation that we can be immersed in suffering and loss daily and not be touched by it is as unrealistic as expecting to be able to walk through water without getting wet' (Remen, 2006). VT is one of the ways walking through water makes us get wet.

In comparison to other forms of workplace trauma, VT occurs beneath consciousness. We don't notice it is happening, and it sneaks into us in various hidden forms. VT occurs from exposure to the trauma of others. It's a relational experience and it is linked to attunement or empathy. VT usually occurs from sustained and repeated empathic engagement with people who have experienced trauma, but this can include so many of our patients. VT alters deep belief systems about safety and trust (in the same way that trauma does). In fact, VT is indistinguishable from a trauma response, but because nothing in particular has happened to us, we may not recognise it as such.

VT occurs as a side effect of empathy, upon which many nursing and midwifery therapeutic relationships are built. Many nursing and midwifery roles require us to use empathic engagement to build therapeutic relationships. Empathy requires projecting ourselves into the experience of others, activating mirror neurons in the brain and other neural pathways which replicate other people's emotional states. This means that when we 'tune into' patients, our brains (to activate empathic feelings) replicate a representation of what we think they are experiencing. This is usual and helpful. However, when this happens over and over again, and especially when we are in workplaces where there is inadequate time to rest and regulate, it makes sense that the wheels start to fall off this process a little. We may, at some level of consciousness, stop being able to identify what experience is ours and what is someone else's. Through replicating the trauma experiences of others to understand them, we start to feel traumatised. This doesn't mean that we believe we have experienced a trauma that we haven't, but it does mean that our attempts to replicate what it feels like to experience trauma can start to be mistaken for our own experiences. This is different from workplace trauma, compassion fatigue, or burnout.

VT occurs gradually, mimics experiences of trauma, and can result in sustained shifts in our perceptions of the world, beneath consciousness. This is different from just being impacted or distressed by our work. It is about how work can change us. For example, a person who works with survivors of traumatic car accidents may, over time, find themselves unable to travel in cars without experiencing their own traumatic symptoms of hyper- or hypo-arousal. In this way, they are experiencing the effects of the trauma of car accidents and may have less trust in the world as a safe place, without ever having experienced an accident directly. This is a relatively straightforward example, but shifts in perceptions of the world due to VT exposure can happen with all sorts of trauma, in subtle and complex ways, across settings. Someone working with women in a sexual assault service who previously dated men may no longer be able to date men. They may not recognise that this shift in how they view and interact with potential partners is linked to their work, but a deep shift has occurred in trust, beliefs, and connection. VT can alter how we relate to our families, loved ones, or our activities of daily living. In the same way that traumatic responses can be understood as 'normal' responses to abnormal situations, VT is a normal reaction to empathic engagement with traumatic material.

VT occurs gradually over time. We don't wake up one day and feel vicariously traumatised. Slowly, beneath consciousness, we may develop altered cognitive schemas of safety, trust, power, and intimacy, such as may occur with interpersonal trauma. Because nothing specific has happened, we won't anchor these experiences to an event. In this way, VT is almost like an intestinal parasite that settles in; it takes something from us without us realising. 'Symptoms' of VT include apathy, exhaustion, irritability, cynicism, and disillusionment, but really the symptoms are as diverse as those of trauma. People may experience distraction, changes in mood or humour, feeling unsafe, increased substance use, decreased sleep, cynicism, memory, negativity, disconnection, loss of purpose and hope, anger, helplessness, confusion, ambivalence, grief, distress, and altered views and beliefs about the world. Like trauma, VT can lead to numbness, fear, rage, sadness, anxiety, depression, helplessness, despair, and shame, as well as fluctuations between numbness and overwhelming emotion. Physiological effects can include sleep disturbance, racing heart, nightmares, loss of appetite, fatigue, irritability, distraction, as well as behavioural effects such as social withdrawal or isolation and instability of other parts of life. Changes in worldview can impact work if we find it hard to engage with some patients or colleagues, or we lose confidence in ourselves and our work.

VT has long been recognised in trauma therapy fields, yet is only beginning to be identified in general healthcare settings. A natural result of increased trauma awareness is that we, as staff, may become more aware of our own personal experiences of trauma. As part of this, it may seem like being more knowledgeable about trauma makes us more susceptible to VT, as we are noticing and talking about trauma more. However, awareness of VT is what allows us to understand it, integrate it, and reduce its impacts, and this requires awareness of trauma.

Addressing vicarious trauma using ABC

Alongside recognising that many nurses and midwives may experience VT, it is important to acknowledge that we also know what helps. All experiences of trauma can feel helpless, like once we are fundamentally changed by something, nothing can be done.

Table 14.1 The ABC of vicarious trauma intervention

Awareness	Awareness of VT is essential for being able to recognise it and understand it. This requires access to education and information, as well as self-reflection. It is important for all nurses and midwives to remain curious about how VT may impact them and establish supportive professional relationships (such as mentors, clinical supervisors, or others) that can help them reflect on any alterations in their worldview or well-being
Balance	It can be difficult to maintain work-life balance in nursing and midwifery due to a lack of staff and resources, rostering, and shift work. Balance in the context of VT may mean ensuring a moment's downtime between patients, taking allocated breaks, ensuring time for positive and fulfilling activities, and opportunities to engage in relationships where you do not take on a caregiving role
Connection	Trauma leads to disconnection. It is important, therefore, to ensure connections are established and maintained prior to experiences of VT, as these can be protective and helpful. Connection refers to people who you regularly talk to about your work and how it impacts you. They can be informal (such as trusted colleagues) or formal (such as employee assistance programmes) and should be people who have an understanding of you and the work that you do, as well as are themselves aware of the risks of VT

Counteracting this helplessness with understandings of recovery and post-traumatic growth is important. For VT, the most significant thing that 'helps' is awareness. The best defence against an unconscious response to transferred trauma is becoming aware of its effects. Like the intestinal worm, once we know it is there or we recognise the risk factors, we can treat it or take preventative action. From knowing, we are left less powerless or confused by its effects. As such, the first step of becoming vicariously trauma informed is knowing about it and talking about it. In the act of recognition of automatic responses, the higher cortical centres, particularly the frontal lobes, are recruited. These integrate and contextualize responses to trauma and provide a basis for its resolution. Following awareness, balance and connection are also needed (see Table 14.1).

I was personally humbled by VT during the pandemic. I was working clinically, working too many hours providing telehealth counselling to distressed pregnant folks while sitting in a windowless office. I started going home feeling overwhelmed, anxious, and not sleeping. I wasn't myself, but then who was at that time? It took me a while to recognise what was happening. It took me a while to see that how I felt was not a reaction to my life but a reflection of the cumulative absorption of the stories I was hearing, without opportunities to separate me from them. The circumstances amplified this; there was a lot of distress, so I felt compelled to book appointments back-to-back. All of the appointments were via telehealth, so I had no visual cues of their being an 'other', and in addition, all of the stories were quite similar. All the clients were women of childbearing age who were pregnant and distressed. I had no way to interrupt the repeated pathways of empathy that were required to do my job well. Over time, I began to take on the helplessness and fear of the women I was caring for and blur it with my own.

Once I realised this, a few things really helped. Firstly, realising itself helped. How I realised it is hard to say. I was actually writing a paper about VT at the time, so you would think I would have seen it coming, but that is not how VT works. It was not until my life started to unravel that I had to stop and really reflect on what was happening.

When I realised what it might have been, my eyes suddenly opened. The most profound thing that happened was that I had a way to understand how I felt. The overwhelming feelings became comprehensible. And I had a way to 'do something' in the face of trauma. I started making small changes to my days – I stepped outside and looked at the sky in between patients to orient myself in time and space, and I scheduled at least 5 minutes between phone calls and used that time intentionally to regulate, tapping my arms and legs to remind myself of the boundaries of me. I started calling a friend on the way home from work, forcing a different relational experience into my day, or I would listen to loud music and lose myself in the sounds. I would shower when I got home to wash the day away. These are small acts that I can imagine people saying they already do or for various reasons aren't possible. But the idea is that you do whatever you can do, and you do it with intention. I essentially developed a routine to separate my self from other people's selves.

At an individual level, strategies are required to buffer against the effects of VT and preserve the sense of self. This may require us to notice shifts and be curious about what might be happening for us. This includes being aware in the moment of clinical encounters, of what is happening with our breathing, sensations, and affect. While being present for our patients, we are also conscious of what is happening in ourselves in response and curious about why. For example, *why does my chest feel tight after I engage with that patient? Why do I feel cranky after I perform this task?*

Looking after each other is also important. This occurs through things like checking in with colleagues, finding trusted colleagues with whom we can intentionally talk about the work, and informally debriefing after events. It can also include accessing clinical supervision, peer support, or workplace assistance programmes. All of these things help us shine a light on what lurks in our shadows. Without these, there is an unconscious temptation to hide how we feel, or to not acknowledge responses to the work, or to build shame around our reactions. It can be difficult to let other people know if we are concerned about them, but finding safe ways within teams to talk about the way the work impacts us is also critical.

Organisations also have a responsibility to protect nurses and midwives from VT. Organisations have responsibilities to ensure fair and manageable workloads, access to supervision, debriefing and support, adequate breaks, and psychological resources for staff. Organisations should also implement preventative and interventional structures including access to information, education, and resources. As part of movements towards being trauma informed, organisations are setting themselves a task to support staff who may be at risk of VT from their work. It is important for nursing and midwifery workplaces to support nurses and midwives to develop ways of talking about and identifying workplace trauma and ensuring access to interventions to help manage the effects within work. We can do what we can to manage ourselves, but it is also about organisational cultures, and ideally it is about prevention.

Not all effects of exposure to other people's trauma are problematic. For many of us, being able to connect with people during difficult moments of their lives is what makes the work rewarding. In the same we may replicate their experiences of trauma through empathy, it is also possible that we may replicate their experiences of resilience and resistance. This can lead to vicarious post-traumatic growth (VPTG). VPTG refers to the positive changes that can occur after indirect exposure to traumatic events. Positive changes can include an enhanced sense of self, richness in relationships, and philosophical sense-making about life. These experiences may not counteract any negative effects or cancel out distress, but they can be concurrent or prominent. Social support, feeling professionally valued, and job satisfaction are correlated with VPTG.

Self-care is a part of trauma informed work

Self-care to manage the effects of VT is essential. Self-care means different things to different people. It can be increased by ensuring access to relaxation activities, reciprocal relationships outside of work, work/life balance, use of positive coping mechanisms, and stress reduction techniques. The principles of trauma intervention are also relevant with a need to ensure safety, connection, processing of experiences, and meaning-making.

Traditional self-care includes any practice or action that preserves or improves health and well-being. Traditional approaches to self-care can be physical (such as sleep, eating well, and preventative healthcare), professional (such as managing boundaries and workload, seeking clinical supervision, and maintaining work-life balance), and personal (maintaining social roles and networks, engaging coping strategies, managing stress, and undertaking intentional, enjoyable activities). One challenge for self-care is that it should be both sustainable and life-enhancing. It requires intentionality to achieve a life pace and flow that is both of these things. This means that self-care isn't more work and emotional labour and something we 'have to do', nor does it symbolically represent 'health' or 'wellbeing' without actually serving the purpose of enabling these experiences. Many nurses and midwives hear the word(s) 'self-care' and may feel it is asking something else of them or is tokenistic in the face of stress and workload.

Self-care can be pushed upon people as something else they have to do, or it can be positioned as an individual obligation amongst social or professional expectation. For example, on occasion workplaces may support staff well-being through discounted gym memberships or lunchtime meditation sessions. While these support staff health, they still require staff to give up their personal time to do more. In addition, people may feel they don't have the time to 'do' self-care or that it should be something that moves them towards health, even if unpleasant or unenjoyable. This isn't how I understand self-care.

Experiences of VT or burnout can feel very isolating and individualised; trauma nearly always isolates people. And the suggested treatment is also nearly always individual counselling, supervision, or self-care. But self-care does not change the contexts in which we work or our patients live, nor does it make those responsible accountable. It is not for people who experience assault to have to work harder to manage ongoing experiences of assault, and it is also not for staff to have to work harder to manage VT in workplaces that continue to perpetrate harm.

Radicalising ideas of self-care

There have long been movements to radicalise ideas of self-care. Radical self-care was driven by the work of feminist women of colour, such as Audre Lorde (Lorde & Sanchez, 2017), who identified that women of colour need to consciously practice self-care and self-love to cope with the daily onslaught of racism, sexism, homophobia, and class oppression. To do so is an act of resistance against structures which exert power and oppress.

Radical self-care requires doing the things that make us feel good. Self-care can be a collective undertaking, embedded in connection and caring. It can also be wild. Wild self-care, as described by Clay (2022), can be messy and based on recovering aspects of the self.

It can encompass things we do to protect ourselves and our well-being (such as cancelling social events or complaining to trusted friends or reaching out for support), things we do to heal and restore ourselves (like swimming in the ocean, listening to punk rock, or spiritual activities), and things that are emancipatory (like rotting in bed, reading fantasy books, or planning holidays). These things exist outside and above the tasks that are essential for maintaining a self – like drinking enough water, sleeping well, and cleaning your space.

Engaging with radicalised politics of self-care is inextricably tied to the lived experiences of people who live with trauma, illness, and disability or are marginalised from mainstream society. This includes people whose bodies don't fit expected norms or whose place in society is tenuous. For example, if a conventionally attractive, slim person enjoys a sweet treat, this could be considered self-care, while if a larger bodied or fat person does it, it may be assumed to be indulgence. Or if a high achieving 'successful' person takes a holiday, it may be considered well-earned self-care, whereas for a less financially secure person or a person of lower social status, it may be seen as frivolous or self-indulgent.

Radicalised ideas of self-care in work combine elements of traditional ideas of self-care (for example, boundary setting and taking your breaks) with elements of activism for change (for example, advocating for nursing and midwifery conditions). It can also mean finding moments of micro-care, if chunks of time is not an available privilege. Self-care should have both professional and personal domains. This requires a commitment to looking after self, in the same way that as nurses and midwives we make a commitment to looking after others.

Finally, I want to note that self-care of any kind is not the antidote to burnout or VT. It is too individualised and does not acknowledge the contexts in which we work. It is not all on us to keep ourselves well. But it is part of our work, and seeing self-care as part of our work is part of being trauma informed.

References

Choi, K. R., Hughesdon, K., Britton, L., Sinko, L., Wells, C., Giordano, N., Sarna, L., & Heilemann, M. V. (2022). Interpersonal trauma in the lives of nurses and perceptions of nursing work. *Western Journal of Nursing Research*, *44*(8), 734–742. https://doi.org/10.1177/01939459211015894

Clay, S. (2022). Wild self-care. *Somatechnics*, *12*(1–2), 73–91. https://doi.org/10.3366/soma.2022.0378

Foli, K. J., Reddick, B., Zhang, L., & Krcelich, K. (2020). Nurses' psychological trauma: "They leave me lying awake at night." *Archives of Psychiatric Nursing*, *34*(3), 86–95. https://doi.org/10.1016/j.apnu.2020.04.011

Hall, L. W., & Scott, S. D. (2012). The second victim of adverse health care events. *Nursing Clinics of North America*, *47*(3), 383–393.https://doi.org/10.1016/j.cnur.2012.05.008

Isobel, S. (2021). Is trauma informed care possible in the current public mental health system?. *Australasian Psychiatry*, *29*(6), 607–610. https://doi.org/10.1177/10398562211028625

Lorde, A., & Sanchez, S. (2017). *A burst of light: And other essays*. Ixia Press.

Remen, R. N. (2006). *Kitchen table wisdom: Stories that heal* (10th anniversary ed.). Riverhead Books.

Sanchez, M., Simon, A., & Ford, D. (2019). PTSD in Tx ICU Nurses. *The Journal of Heart and Lung Transplantation*, *38*(4), S93–S94. https://doi.org/10.1016/j.healun.2019.01.217

Saunders, B. E., & Adams, Z. W. (2014). Epidemiology of traumatic experiences in childhood. *Child and Adolescent Psychiatric Clinics of North America*, *23*(2), 167–184. https://doi.org/10.1016/j.chc.2013.12.003

15 Considerations for trauma informed care implementation

When I first started thinking about trauma informed care (TIC) and trying to spread the ideas, I discovered that implementation was never easy. To me, TIC makes sense, and I expected that others would also be immediately on board with the approach. I was wrong. Implementing TIC is a transformative process that requires a comprehensive and thoughtful approach. Trauma informed practice takes time and ideally requires significant involvement from others and a team approach. However, even if this isn't possible, all nurses and midwives can implement TIC within their own practice on an everyday basis to improve outcomes for their patients and themselves.

Implementing trauma informed care

To implement TIC within services, nurses and midwives need time to learn about trauma from knowledgeable people, and to understand its relevance to their context of work. Alongside any generic training, nurses and midwives require time and space to discuss what TIC means in their practice, in their setting, and with their clients. In addition, all nurses and midwives need access to referral pathways and information about available local services to refer people and support to figure out how to identify, document, and talk about trauma safely. Nurses and midwives need opportunities to practice using regulation to manage distress and they need access to resources that support grounding and co-regulation. Nurses and midwives need motivation to change their individual practice, alongside policies and leadership that demonstrate wider commitments to change.

Sometimes people feel that they have always been trauma informed in their practice and that TIC is just a new way to describe their usual practice. While this may be true in some instances, there is also a risk of mistaking the outcomes of trauma informed ways of practising with having the depth of knowledge about trauma that guides these outcomes. For example, we can all perform the tasks of washing our hands and wearing masks which can give the impression of infection control and can also be largely effective. However, if we don't understand how infections spread, then we can't be flexible enough to account for the need to have your nose covered by the mask, to not touch the outside of the mask, to notice when someone is showing symptoms of illness, to know when the right moments are to wash our hands, to know the importance of soap and drying hands, and so on. Similarly, we can take people's vital signs accurately and carefully, and document them correctly, but unless we have knowledge of what they are telling us about the body and the person's health, we may not interpret the overall picture correctly. The same is true of TIC. It is possible to provide care in ways that make

DOI: 10.4324/9781003530770-18

people feel safe and allow for choice and trust without having knowledge of trauma. But to be trauma informed requires an understanding of trauma that then guides our practice. When we understand trauma, we are responsive in the moment to what may be happening for someone and why.

When I was working in an acute mental health inpatient unit that was implementing TIC, often people would want to come and 'see' the trauma informed unit. This always made me nervous. While the unit was structurally very nice and had trauma informed considerations in the availability of spaces, sensory items, and information, most TIC is invisible. It is built into how staff interact with people, how decisions are made, and how people are thought about and talked about. Some of these things can be 'seen', but the thinking and knowledge that underpins them (that is, the knowledge of trauma which informs care) is not visible. TIC can look like basic good practice, but the meaning is in the details of how it makes people feel.

Steps for implementation

When I first started 'implementing' TIC in a conscious way, it was to use it as a nursing model of care on one acute inpatient unit. In hindsight, this was not ideal. It doesn't make sense to have one trauma informed unit. It implies that it is a choice, when in fact it is an organisational approach that should include all parts of a service. It needs to involve implementation processes, training for staff, opportunities for staff reflection, policy and procedures, and plans for reviewing little bits of practice and big bits of practice. Over the years, I have learnt that having plans and checklists is helpful and making sure there are ongoing opportunities to talk about trauma is essential. I have also learnt that there is a need to be trauma informed in the process of change. This means modelling the principles of how change is implemented so that staff can stay engaged in the process.

Questions and prompts to support implementation

There are a lot of implementation tools freely available to support structured organisational approaches to TIC. These are very useful, but this is not that. These are lists to help you think through aspects of TIC and to provide guidance if you are feeling stuck.

Individual practice improvement

Sometimes the best place to start is with ourselves. Often, once we engage with information about trauma, we feel ready to start being trauma informed, but it is not always clear how to begin. These prompts may be helpful in identifying starting points.

- Seek out education and information about trauma (there are lots of free and available videos and courses, plus there may be some already within your workplace). Think about what trauma may mean for the people you provide care to.
- Listen to, or read, the experiences of people who have accessed your type of service – what do they describe?
- Consider the aspects of your practice or service that you feel discomfort about and consider why. What aspects of these could be altered?
- Notice how people respond to you at work (and consider why).

- Notice how work makes you feel (and consider why).
- Notice which clients or patients activate irritation, distress, or concern in you (and consider why).
- Notice how you speak about people who access your service – is the focus on what is wrong with them medically? Is there an opportunity to consider more about their life and circumstances?
- Consider how others may experience you, what feeling or vibe do you give off? Is there a way to take a moment to regulate yourself prior to any interaction to enable therapeutic presence?
- Consider the spaces in which you engage with people – what can be seen, heard, or smelled? These things can't always be altered, but they can be acknowledged.
- What choices are offered or possible in how people engage with you?
- Consider the social, political, and structural context of your local environment and catchment area. What may contribute to people's experiences of trauma or adversity?
- How do you greet people in the clinical context – are there opportunities to be more trustworthy in how you introduce yourself?
- Notice how you stand or sit, what you hold, and what you do with your face, body, and voice when you interact with patients. Are there cues of power and/or cues of safety?
- How do patients access you if they need something? How accessible is this process?
- Are there points in care that may be more likely to activate shame? What can you do to be shame sensitive?
- If a patient disclosed trauma to you, what would you do? What would you say? Who would you refer to?
- What could you say to yourself or do to regulate yourself if you were becoming hypo- or hyper-aroused in the clinical context?
- How do you feel after work? What are the things that stay with you? What can you do to separate your work self from your home self?
- What opportunities for reflection do you have, either with others (through supervision, debriefing, or peer support) or privately (through journalling, talking to loved ones, or spending time thinking and making sense of things)
- How do you look after yourself during and after work?

Noticing trauma

Part of being trauma informed is noticing. This includes noticing how people engage with your service or care and considering the possibility that trauma may play a role in people's difficulties engaging or the ways they engage. There are likely unique ways that trauma shows up in your settings. These prompts may just help you start to think about what they are.

Have you noticed:

- Frequent cancellation of appointments or failure to show up
- Agitation in waiting areas
- Heightened emotions or responses ('big' responses in the present)
- Lack of emotion or responses
- Startle reflexes or flinches when touched
- Non-verbal cues or disconnections
- Lack of cohesion in history or narration of events

- Emotion without explanation or even awareness
- Signs of physiological arousal such as heightened heart or breathing rate, tone, or rate of speech
- Interactions that leave you feeling confused or frustrated

None of these factors are diagnostic of trauma. They may just be clues and prompts for you to consider moments that may require you to be more trauma sensitive. It is also helpful to notice how you and your colleagues respond to different patients. Noticing how we feel in connection with patients and considering what might be happening for them and for you 'in the moment' can be a clue.

Self-reflection

Trauma and engaging vicariously with trauma pull us away from ourselves and the present. Part of our therapeutic engagement as nurses and midwives is working to be intentionally present. To achieve this requires ongoing self-reflection. The following questions may be helpful to hold in mind as you go about our work. They can also be useful in clinical supervision.

Before interactions with patients

- Am I present and engaged? Where is my mind?
- What is getting in the way of connection for me today?
- What am I hoping for in this interaction? What are the essential things that need to be achieved? How can I clearly communicate what I need from the patient?
- What do I know about this person and their life? What would it be helpful to know that I don't yet know?

During interactions with patients

- What can I do to make this person feel safer?
- What choices are possible?
- How trustworthy am I being?
- Can we collaborate more?
- How can I share power with them?
- What symbols of power am I displaying?
- Could I ask them what they need from me or what might help to make them feel more comfortable?
- Am I listening more than I am talking (excluding the delivery of essential information)?
- How can I steer them towards safety (for example, to private spaces if talking about private things, or validating but pausing topics that cannot be safely discussed)?
- How can I end this conversation in a way that leaves them feeling heard and clear on next steps?

After interactions with patients

- How might that person have experienced that interaction with me?
- What might have happened to this person in their life that has led them to respond to me in this way?

- In what ways may I have signalled power in the interaction?
- What cues did I miss of connection or disconnection?
- Were there any ruptures? Were these repaired either directly or indirectly?
- What vulnerability or need may behaviours be defending against (and how can we help them with this)?
- What is important to document? Am I using words and phrases that are respectful and empowering?

Trauma informed responses for difficult moments

Being trauma informed is not always easy, and it doesn't always go smoothly. When things don't go well, scanning the environment may help, along with systematically thinking through each principle. These questions may also help.

- What assumptions do I bring to my work about patients and their experiences?
- Is there any way I could attempt to make this person feel safer at this moment?
- Am I regulated within myself? What is my body, voice, face, or demeanour communicating?
- Are there any environmental factors which may be making this person feel unsafe?
- Am I triggered myself? Can I slow my breathing, feel my feet on the ground, and return to the present?
- Can I validate their experience or try to name their emotion?
- Are there any feasible or possible choices I can offer?
- Am I being as trustworthy as I can be (being upfront, honest, genuine, and doing all the things I said I would do)?
- Is there any way I could share my power with this person through information, action, or conversation?
- Have I provided meaningful opportunities for this person to collaborate on the plan?
- Could this be a way this person interacts in their wider life? What purpose may this serve?
- How might people usually respond to this person?
- Is the discomfort I feel theirs or mine?
- Am I able to tolerate silence or distress?
- How would it be to narrate my uncertainty about what this person needs and seek suggestions from them?
- What opportunities do I have to debrief or reflect on this interaction with a trusted colleague?

Team or service level implementation of trauma informed care

If possible, it is always a good idea to engage more with the context you work in. Consider finding allies who are also interested in starting from a stance of curiosity. The following questions may be helpful to collaboratively consider:

- Have you consulted widely across your team, service, or organisation (including with people who may be obstructive or who hold unofficial power in teams)?
- Have you considered establishing a working group or committee with multi-level representation and a fair opportunity for anyone to join?

- Is there a way to seek organisational level buy-in (you will need this to make any changes and to ensure sustainability)?
- Is it possible to meaningfully engage Lived Experience representatives or include the voices of patients and their families in working towards TIC?
- Have you considered the use of a structured audit or implementation tool?
- Have you considered the scope of your implementation – is this about nursing and midwifery, or is it multidisciplinary?
- Does everyone have the same understanding of what trauma means in your context? Is it possible to write it down and consult on it?
- Do you have a shared vision of what 'trauma informed' might look like in your setting? Can you write it down and stick it on a noticeboard, giving people opportunities to add to the vision?
- Do you have a plan? A written plan should evolve with the process, but it will be helpful to keep track of any actions or parts. TIC can rapidly become everything and nothing without a plan.
- What opportunities are there for education about trauma for staff – this can be short in-services or longer training programmes, but all staff should have an opportunity to attend. Is it possible to consider rolling or ongoing opportunities to talk about trauma?
- Are there opportunities in the structure of the day for staff to reflect on practice and learnings? These can be formal sessions or brief collegial opportunities, but they are important and should be regular and supported.
- Could a few people audit the environment? How does it feel to enter the service? What are the first things people might notice or feel? How does it feel to leave?
- What are the organisational or service barriers to change? Why do these things exist? What is possible to influence?
- Who are the people least on board with TIC? How could you engage them more or provide opportunities to hear about their reservations?
- Can you consider opportunities to support or advocate for workforce well-being? This may include supervision, adequate breaks and workloads, education about vicarious trauma, and clear pathways to the employee support programme, but first ask people what they need.
- Is it possible to track patient journeys through your service or unit and identify opportunities (or touch points) for improvement?
- Is it possible to reflect on the details of practices that are considered to be 'already trauma informed' – what are the things that make them so, what is noticeable, and what can be learned from these?
- Who is best placed to review policies and procedures through a trauma informed lens? What is the process to make any changes?
- What local trauma-specific services and resources exist that can be provided to patients?
- What mechanisms of feedback and ongoing review could help you evaluate and sustain efforts towards TIC?

Trauma informed documentation

The way nurses and midwives talk about our patients when they aren't around can indicate how we think about people. While we all may complain about our work sometimes or need to 'debrief' about a difficult interaction or situation, it is part of our professionalism and humanity to talk about people with respect and to use words we wouldn't mind them hearing us say about them. This is also true of documentation.

Often, we document defensively. In mental health nursing, for example, we are taught to document in ways that will stand up in court. This leads us to write things like 'patient reported…' or 'patient allegedly experienced….' Or 'patient claims to have experienced…'. We may also go so far as to weave in some epistemic injustice through questioning their reality, for example, by documenting that we saw no evidence of something that they say they experienced or by reporting their experience alongside an assessment of their symptoms. This is invalidating and feeds into ideas that people fictitiously report experiences of abuse. It is trauma un-informed.

There is a way to document that can meet our legal requirements and fears, but still be trauma informed. Documentation about people carries power, and in being conscious of power, our documentation should centre the person and their needs. In a healthcare context, this means considering how we describe people, their experiences, and their behaviours. One way to think about this is to focus on describing what might be happening for the person rather than what they are doing. It can be a subtle shift in language, but it is important in promoting agency and sharing power (Box 15.1).

Box 15.1: Examples of trauma informed documentation

Trauma un-informed documentation	*Trauma informed alternative*
Patient became rude during showering, verbally aggressive towards nurses	The process of showering triggered distress for patient who expressed verbal agitation and declined help from nurses
Patient appears highly sensitive to pain, demanding pain relief and refusing alternative strategies	Patient expressing pain and requesting pain relief. Does not find alternate strategies helpful
Patient difficult to engage	Nursing attempts to engage with patient were ineffective
Patient manipulative of nurses, frequently pressing the buzzer overnight and refusing redirection	Patient experiencing frequent and sustained distress overnight. Frequent calls for assistance from nurses, finds alternate suggestions for soothing not useful
Unable to determine dilation as the patient refusing internal examination	Dilation not currently known as patient prefers not to have internal examinations

Wright and Laurent write about 'trauma informed archiving' (see Wright & Laurent, 2021), recognising that archival work is about memory. They reflect on the importance that comes with being tasked with documenting and storing collective and individual memories, and the need to hold collaboration, empowerment, and safety in mind when doing so that archival work can enact justice doing and healing. The same is true of health records and documentation. Health records both create and document trauma, storing details of people's intimate lives and bodies. When people access their files under

Freedom of Information laws and similar, experiences of trauma can be compounded by what they read about themselves, be it judgemental, through an expert lens, dehumanising, or missing the point. I have sat with many people as they read over the documentation of their labour and delivery of their baby and observed their distress from the absence of humanity. They feel that their pain, their wishes, and their acts of resistance or strength are lost in the cold factual documentation. Conversely, I have sat with a friend while she read her medical records from a psychiatric admission, where she was outraged at how they described her every move, what she was wearing, and how she was acting and used it as 'evidence' of her insanity. We reflected on how our everyday appearances (which are always scruffy) could be used against us. Medical records, like archives, are sites of power.

Trauma informed nursing and midwifery education

Being trauma informed extends beyond clinical care. If you are delivering education in the clinical setting or other professional settings, this is another space to consider being trauma informed. The power dynamics of training and education can activate shame for many people, and there is a need to actively ensure safety within the teaching space and with the way content is delivered. In delivering any nursing and midwifery education, you may want to consider the principles of TIC in relation to what you present and how. The following prompts may help.

Safety

- Do participants know what is expected of them in relation to participation?
- Have you prioritised safety and trust in the space and in your engagement?
- Have you given participants a content overview that will allow them to prepare themselves for any potential triggers?
- Have you scrutinised the language you are using when talking about patients, families, and communities? Are there any misuses of power minimised?
- How will you support the use of safe storytelling in the session?

Choice

- Do participants have a choice about attending the session? If it is mandatory, acknowledge the discomfort this can cause.
- Pay attention to minimising shaming behaviours in the delivery. This includes not putting people on the spot or setting people up.
- Have you accounted for the possibility that your audience or students may also have experienced the conditions you are talking about and minimised the use of 'othering' language?

Collaboration

- Consider how to support all participants to express their opinions and ideas while not allowing violence to occur in the teaching space; this may involve clear establishment of group expectations (for example, 'try not to cut other people off but there may be times when I step in to ensure that the conversation remains safe and collaborative') and practising a sentence you could use to interrupt if tensions get high (for example, 'I am just going to stop you there for a moment to check in with the group').

- How will you make space for everyone in the session to participate?
- Have you scheduled any time or structure after the session to enable you to debrief with a trusted colleague?
- Have you included ways to gather useful and anonymous feedback from participants.

Empowerment

- Do participants know what is acceptable in relation to interrupting, leaving, or taking a break from the session?
- Will you be ready to advocate for individuals or groups should any microaggressions occur during the session?
- Have you left time for participants to ask questions and share reflections?

Trustworthiness

- Have you established a few minutes before the session to ensure you are present and engaged?
- Is the content readily linkable to the intent of the session?
- If teaching directly about trauma informed ideas, ensure you do not present it as a checklist of activities, but leave space for flexibility and adaptation.
- Have you made time to reflect on how engaged and attentive participants were and to use this to inform your ongoing refinement?

Box 15.2: Do trigger warnings work?

Trigger warnings have been taken up across settings. These are usually a statement prior to a lecture, a show, a story, or a social media post that outlines what potential triggers may be included or warns that there may be distressing content. Trigger warnings are intended to keep people safe and signal awareness of trauma. However, research has found that trigger warnings don't seem to result in a decrease in distress and can at times cause distress through anticipation. For example, if you hear that a talk is going to involve details of something distressing, you may feel stressed waiting for the distressing material to be discussed, playing out in your mind what it may include, and essentially thinking of all the triggering things you can while you wait. When embedded as part of a broader trauma informed approach, trigger warnings may be helpful in providing people with opportunities to prepare themselves and look after themselves, but relying solely on trigger warnings, without a wider context of trauma awareness, likely does more harm than good.

There are a few reasons I am not a fan of trigger warnings. The first is that they reinforce the idea that what 'triggers' people is obvious and avoidable. What triggers people can be complex dynamics or a way of being or a smell or a sound. It is an assumption of power to think we know how to prevent all triggers. I also don't like that they can be used to imply awareness of trauma, without actually being aware of trauma, or that they position people who experience trauma as vulnerable or volatile. But I do like letting people know what to expect. And I do like people feeling safe. An alternative is using a content overview rather than a trigger warning. A content overview is always helpful for anyone, regardless of whether they have a history of trauma or not. We would all like to know what will be discussed, and telling people what won't be discussed is also helpful. Mostly people prefer to know what you are doing to keep them safe rather than having to be prepared to keep themselves safe based on the material you will cover. For example, you might say, 'this lecture will not include specific details of any experiences of abuse or neglect' or 'this next slide includes a photo of a person who has been assaulted'. In this, the audience can be emotionally prepared and empowered to make their own decisions about engagement. Minimising sharing of unnecessary details is also trauma informed. There are only a few situations where sharing actual details of terrible things happening to people is necessary, admittedly some of which are in healthcare contexts.

Trauma informed nursing and midwifery research

Nursing and midwifery research often engages with participants or communities who have experienced trauma. Much nursing and midwifery research focuses on sensitive topics or evaluates processes of care that may have been traumatising. Research processes also have the potential to replicate power dynamics that can be reminiscent of trauma. It is therefore important to be trauma informed in undertaking research (Isobel, 2021; Isobel et al., 2024). While being trauma informed involves working through the principles 'in the moment', as it does in clinical and educational settings, it also requires consideration of knowledge of trauma in how studies are designed, undertaken, and disseminated. The following questions may help prompt reflection.

Safety

- Have you considered how you will protect participants, data, and communities from harm during and after the research?
- How prepared do you feel to be able to respond to distress in ways that support people to stay engaged and feel validated?
- How will you maintain your own safety and well-being throughout this work?
- Do you feel confident in identifying cues of engagement, disengagement, dissociation, and distress?

Choice

- Have you provided as many opportunities as possible for people to choose whether they want to engage in the study?
- Can you ensure people have a choice about which questions or components they participate in (this includes making sure questions on surveys are not mandatory)?

Collaboration

- Have you identified which conversations are important to have in the development and undertaking of this study?
- How will you manage the duality of roles as a researcher and also a nurse or midwife?
- What mechanisms of dissemination may ensure findings provide benefit to the communities and individuals?

Empowerment

- Is power shared in the processes of this study?
- Who is defining the vulnerability of the participants and has this been addressed in a transparent way that also promotes agency?
- Have you considered who will benefit from this research?
- Have you reflected on your own positionality within the study?

Trustworthiness

- Have you clearly articulated the intent and outputs of this research?
- Are participants aware of all the ways you will use and analyse their data?
- Have you taken the time to consider what may be impacting participants' experiences, words, or responses and your understanding of them?
- In research about trauma, are you being careful not to conflate the event with the effect? For example, avoid using tools such as the ACE score as a 'measure' of trauma.
- Are you prepared enough that you are able to focus on the participant rather than just the process?
- Do you know where to seek help if you need it?

To be trauma informed requires ongoing vigilance, self-reflection, and collaboration. There are numerous tools and systematic approaches to implementation and lots of places to start. There is also no perfect way to start. It can be helpful to think, talk to people, find allies, start to notice things, and go from there. In any implementation process, it is also important to start slowly and be as trauma informed as you can in the process, with yourself and others.

References

Isobel, S. (2021). Trauma-informed qualitative research: Some methodological and practical considerations. *International Journal of Mental Health Nursing, 30*(S1), 1456–1469. https://doi.org/10.1111/inm.12914

Isobel, S., Clay, S., Sam, K., Jurcevic, C., & Kemp, H. (2024). *Towards trauma-informed research: A brief overview and practice guide.* https://cmhdaresearchnetwork.com.au/resource/towards-trauma-informed-research-a-brief-overview-and-practice-guide/

Wright, K., & Laurent, N. (2021). Safety, collaboration, and empowerment: Trauma-informed archival practice. *Archivaria, 91*, 38–73. https://doi.org/10.7202/1078465ar

16 Moving forward with trauma informed care

There is a pacing to engaging with ideas that must be respected. It takes people time to engage with concepts that are difficult, and it takes time to feel comfortable with uncomfortable things. Even for people who have lived or are living experiences of trauma, there is time needed to engage with the significance of what this means on a systemic level. Some nurses and midwives may already be deep in the politics of trauma, but for many, nursing and midwifery may not always have felt like political spaces. Nurses and midwives are positioned as almost apolitical, able to provide care to anyone and hold back their personal opinions. We strike for better conditions, but we always make sure patients will be cared for while we are gone. We unionise about workloads, but we still do overtime to ensure people don't die. As professionals we are political, but also often careful.

Yet, as humans, once we see something like trauma, it is hard to unsee. We might look at our own lives differently or our relationships differently. We might initially think we have no experience of something and then start to realise we do. We might look at people around us and ourselves differently; we might become hyper aware of things that do not fit or align with what we are thinking about. We can start to get angry at people who don't get it, or we think are blind to it, or at systems or groups who cause harm.

After a while of thinking about what it means to be trauma informed, it can become a struggle to work towards it in systems and services that aren't. Yet it is also a struggle to change systems and services. A few times I have felt unsure if I am driving change within systems that perpetuate harm, or if I am simply part of the system and therefore complicit in harm.

How to keep on keeping on

Despite the challenges, sustaining efforts towards being trauma informed is largely motivated by the inherent knowing we all have of what a difference it can make to our days, experiences, or even lives, to encounter someone who makes us feel safe. For someone to be a nurse or midwife in a healthcare institution where we may feel unsafe can be a hugely impactful experience. Focusing on the relational importance of this is one way to keep on keeping on. Despite the systems and structures, we can refine our own practice to be as sensitive and responsive to trauma as we can. This also requires looking after ourselves. Engaging self-care and preventing vicarious trauma are not additional to being trauma informed; they are imperative and part of the work and should be addressed with due diligence and care.

DOI: 10.4324/9781003530770-19

Another way to keep on is to find allies. It can be unsustainable to become trauma informed on your own. In line with knowledge of trauma, we know that trauma leads to a sense of isolation and a key part of healing is connection. This should also be modelled in the doing. This requires us to find people and allies who also want to work in this way and connect to them. This is essential for sustaining the work. Sustaining trauma informed-ness also requires ongoing engagement with knowledge. Knowledge of trauma is evolving, and our understanding should also. Gaining knowledge of trauma requires us to share that knowledge with others, lest it become another weapon of power. In this way, keeping on requires ongoing engagement and thinking around what it continues to mean to be trauma informed in any context.

Once ideas of trauma in individuals and in individual relationships have marinated, there is a common shifting to the need to consider the wider context of why trauma is so prevalent. This transition takes time and can't be rushed. If we just focus on the systems, then individual experiences can be invalidated or missed. But after seeing repeated individual experiences, there is often a natural consideration of 'why'. It is here that I have found being 'violence informed' at the same time as being 'trauma informed' helpful.

Being trauma and violence informed at once

Being trauma *and violence* informed requires us to consider both the impact of trauma upon the lives of individuals and also the wider context in which this occurs. Through this dual perspective, we concurrently recognise people's individual experiences and hold awareness of the systems of structural violence that have contributed to them. Structural violence refers to systems and processes that systematically disadvantage individuals or populations, increasing risk of harm and perpetuating inequities, often embedded within historical and current social, economic, and political systems. Unlike acts of physical violence, structural violence is often continuous and embedded in societal organisations. While not all experiences of trauma occur in the context of structural violence, for many groups and individuals they do. When I first heard of the idea of trauma and violence informed care, I was unsure about the need to expand the already complex concept of TIC to include structural violence, but I have come to see that this shift to holding both trauma and structures which cause, sustain, and replicate it is important for recognising both historical and ongoing violence, for understanding why some people or groups experience disproportionate amounts or impacts of trauma, and also considering why people may not speak up or act in the moment or aftermath of trauma. It can also help with understanding why things that are set up or done with the best intentions within systems may not be helpful. To use a simple example, perhaps someone sets up a service for people who have experienced trauma, but they hire a space that used to be a church to run it. People may not attend the service, and it can be assumed that people who experienced trauma 'didn't want it', when in fact the space it was in represented a context where people may have experienced harm or mistrust. Similarly, we might wonder why women 'don't just report' their experiences of violence to the police, without recognising how systems like the police can also enact violence and represent masculinity and power. We can misunderstand actions that people do protectively if we focus just on the action and don't turn our eyes to what they are trying to protect against. In addition, we might provide care to people who seem to have a disproportionate amount of hardship or reactions to experiences in their lives. If we don't understand the ways their experiences are silenced, ignored, or reinforced throughout society, then we may not really understand their individual experiences at all. How we consider both trauma and violence in practice is challenging, but reflection is a useful starting point. If trauma informed care requires us to consider 'what might be happening for, or has happened to, this person', then trauma and violence informed care requires us to ask 'why'. This also requires us to consider what role we or our service may play in replicating harm or pathologising individuals.

The shift of the trauma informed care movement into health services has tapped into a deeper philosophical issue around whose responsibility social disadvantage is and where responsibility lies for overcoming adversity. We may not always realise this when we start dabbling in knowledge of trauma, but to be truly trauma informed requires us to engage in the politics of it and to recognise historic and ongoing ways that systems disadvantage people based on class, race, gender, politics, sexuality, beliefs, or other divides. This includes the politics of which groups and individuals have been privileged or protected. To be trauma and violence informed thus requires us to recognise that no amount of privilege can protect humans from the harm that humans can cause in relationship to each other, but that privilege may impact how we access or receive help or assistance. For example, while as nurses or midwives we may have overcome (or continue to survive) enormous hardships in our lives or families, in our work we are holding power and privilege based on our access to education, employment, and knowledge. This may set us, however uncomfortably, apart from people who don't have such access.

Being trauma and violence informed requires us to have knowledge of the pervasive nature of forms of violence, how it can be woven into dynamics of control and power, how it can be accepted, endorsed, or hidden within our communities, and how it is also perpetuated by positioning people who experience it as weak or vulnerable or somehow to blame. Then we have the capacity to respond to individual trauma in a way that recognises the importance of not replicating these same dynamics within our care or framing of the person.

I recall when someone who had spoken out about sexual abuse died by suicide. She had accused someone high profile and powerful of sustained abuse. The claims had been denied. The general public got involved with their own opinions and she received large amounts of scrutiny and criticism. Her life was complex; she had substance use issues and was framed by the media as 'troubled'. There is a way to look at this situation which perpetuates harm, where people's disclosures are disbelieved and their reliability as a witness is questioned. In this framing, power is used against the person who experienced trauma to discredit them and to question their truthfulness. This is the easiest way, and it is what perpetrators and systems of structural violence rely on. There is also another way to look at this, where her hardship and adversity are seen as effects of trauma, sympathy or empathy may be evoked, and some understanding may be generated that her life was unravelled by abuse, leading to substance use and challenges, and that eventually trauma overwhelmed her capacity to cope. To look at this situation through a trauma and violence informed lens requires us to hold awareness of all these dynamics at once: to know that violence is enabled by power which disguises it and by targeting people who have less power or whose power can be eroded. To know that violence likely caused trauma for her and then trauma was sustained by ongoing structural violence which facilitated disbelief, invalidation, and likely fear. I imagine she experienced fear and betrayal by the initial abuse and then she experienced ongoing and compounding fear and betrayal by the world's response to her disclosure.

Some questions to ask yourself in starting to become trauma and violence informed in nursing and midwifery care are: what historical or ongoing disadvantages do people in the communities you provide care to face, how might social or political contexts impact upon people's individual experiences of trauma, what structural or systemic factors impede people's capacity to recover, where are you placed in relation to power and privilege, how do you or your service position individual impacts of trauma as 'the problem', how does your service fit in relation to historical or ongoing harms, how might your service inadvertently disempower people who have experienced trauma and what power dynamics are replicated in care. While these questions may sound overwhelming, thinking in this way has given me a way to 'move forward' with thinking about trauma in the lives of people who access care. Another action we can take if we are unsure how to proceed with trauma and violence informed care is to be curious and open, and ask people what they need: 'are there ways we can make you feel more comfortable while you are here?' or 'are there things it would be helpful for me to know about you?' This allows us to balance respecting the autonomy of people to make decisions about what they share of themselves and being conscious of people not having to articulate everything for us to be sensitive to possibilities.

Our responsibility in being trauma and violence informed extends beyond the individuals we provide direct care to. For example, it can require us to use our position as healthcare workers to stand up for people who have less power when we witness them being harmed. Perhaps we observe our colleagues treating students badly or talking about patients in ways that are degrading. While we may not be actively impacted by what we observe, we are still affected by the power relations it reinforces. Power is not as straightforward as one person or group asserting it over another; it occurs in a context. It can be hard to stand up to misuses of power all the time, and sometimes it isn't safe to do so. But we can do our best to support other people or advocate, we can do things in the moment to signal our beliefs and solidarity, and we can connect with others to work towards advocacy and change.

Working with resistance

When discussing the impacts of childhood trauma on health, Dr Nadine Burke-Harris (Burke-Harris, 2015) describes how she started to understand trauma and got all excited about the implications for her work in paediatrics and wanted to tell her colleagues about it. She says: 'I thought everyone would be on board – but why aren't they?' I have asked myself this same question a lot. Along the way of trying to become more trauma informed, I have encountered a lot of apathy and dismissal. But I have also encountered active resistance. There is, therefore, Nadine's question of why this occurs, and there is a question that somebody asked me recently, which is 'how do you respond?'

There are various answers to why trauma informed approaches activate resistance. In healthcare contexts, change is a constant. Staff get tired of being asked to do more with less, and to implement every new approach while also meeting the demands of their roles. This accounts for everyday resistance to change that we encounter anytime there is a new system, policy, or procedure. But there is something extra about trauma. It activates people's discomfort. Resistance arises from misunderstandings of what being trauma informed means, assumptions of what or who it includes or excludes, over-simplification, over-complication, focusing too much on individuals, or not focusing enough on individuals. When I first started implementing TIC, I was surprised by the resistance and the diverse arguments that went with it. In implementing it into an acute mental health unit, we observed: 'There were paradoxical criticisms that argued that TIC was simultaneously too controversial and too simplistic and there were misunderstandings about the intent of the approach based upon its name. The use of the word "trauma" was seemingly emotive and open to misinterpretation. Some nurses reported feeling criticised, as though their current approach was being labelled traumatising, while others feared the lack of safety that could arise from changes to long-standing practice' (Isobel & Edwards, 2017).

These days, I think resistance is expected whenever power is challenged. Ideas of trauma challenge power and the status quo within social structures and dominant paradigms of understanding health, illness, and recovery. Whenever there are shifts in how we understand or do things, there is resistance. There are also specific aspects of TIC that raise defensiveness. It can feel like a criticism or an attack. It is deeply confronting to consider the harm that can be caused by humans to other humans and the legacy this leaves. It is even more confronting when this occurs in the process of giving or receiving care. Therefore, some resistance to TIC comes from staff feeling attacked or blamed for things that feel unfair or messy.

When I think about how I respond to resistance, I think about the energy that resistance brings. In the same way that we recognise resistance as a part of trauma, it is also a part of change. It has been much harder in my career to respond to apathy than to resistance. Resistance gives a spark and something to discuss. It is actually quite difficult to fundamentally disagree about trauma; we can disagree about who gets to claim legitimacy, we can disagree about responsibility and required actions, we can disagree about what is acceptable to call trauma, and we can disagree about the framing of trauma knowledge. But it is very hard to disagree that some people experience horrid things and are impacted by these.

All nurses, midwives, and healthcare workers can recognise how sometimes the situations we find the most tricky to navigate are with those people who mistrust services, react strongly to attempts to provide care, or seem to have long-standing complex relationships with seeking and receiving care. We can all also recognise that sometimes people react in ways we don't expect to pain, illness, care, and treatment, and there may be things in their lives that help make sense of this. If we can strip back ideas to these shared experiences, there is an opportunity to work together to think about how this understanding impacts care. Some of the best allies I have formed over the years have been people who I didn't initially see eye to eye with. I recall a junior doctor who got into a serious disagreement with a nurse about trauma informed care. He felt it was unsafe and dangerous for nurses to be thinking about or talking about trauma with people who were unwell. It caused a lot of tension. And yet years later, I met that doctor in a different context and he was advocating for less coercive care and de-pathologising experiences. We realised our ideas were aligned all along, but he had reacted strongly to nurses implementing TIC as he felt the blame was being shifted to him. He had a different understanding of what TIC meant, and this led to a defensiveness that meant he couldn't stop to hear. I think I was less patient in those early days with people who showed resistance. Over time, I have learned that these aren't people we should ignore or not worry about; these are the people we need to engage the most.

When dealing with resistance, I also reflect on the commonality I may share with the resistors. To me, trauma informed care is a resistance. It is an act of resistance against dehumanised ways of providing care, resistance against the loss of rights and safety in care, resistance against systemic violence and disadvantages, resistance against lack of care for workforces and workers, and resistance against simplified approaches to complex problems. Maybe within whatever activates resistance in the people who resist trauma informed care, there is some commonality that can be found. Maybe they resist because they have ideas that are uncomfortable, or maybe they are burnt-out or tired, maybe they resist because they think it's another simplified solution to a complex problem, and maybe they resist because they don't yet understand trauma or because they themselves are traumatised. In all these spaces, there is opportunity.

One simple but useful strategy I have held onto is using the principles of TIC in everything that I do. I am no longer just trauma informed in my nursing practice; I am trauma informed in my teaching and research, I am trauma informed in how I try to run meetings or manage my team, and I am trauma informed in how I respond to people who disagree. And I am trauma informed in how I talk about being trauma informed. I am not perfect at this. I'm sure people who know me can think of many times I haven't succeeded in this. But I try. Being trauma informed in introducing ideas of trauma means trying: trying to be attuned to what happens in the moment, noticing shifts in arousal, prioritising safety, not blaming people for their responses, and positioning myself in a space of trying to foster safety, choice, collaboration, empowerment, and trustworthiness in the way that I am going about things. In considering any proposed change to the way care is delivered as a 'threat', I therefore need to consider how I talk about change in ways that make it safe enough for people to be able to hear the messages. How much choice do people who will be impacted have in what is being suggested? How transparent have I been about my agenda? How much opportunity is there to hear about their experiences and perspectives? How psychologically safe do people feel in hearing about trauma and understanding the implications? What might impact this? How much control do they have over what happens? Without this approach, efforts towards TIC can lead to conflict, staff turnover, or resistance.

The limitations and possibilities of trauma informed care

There are risks associated with becoming trauma informed. In my career, I have faced resistance, defensiveness, and outrageous aggression. I have seen staff harmed by attempts to lead its implementation from encountering unexpected hostility and ad hominem defensiveness. I've seen being 'trauma informed' become performative, where services, teams, or individuals identify themselves as being trauma informed for the purposes of appearing progressive or beneficent or safe, without critical reflection on whether this is accurate and also without recognising the dynamic nature of these states. I have been actively committed to trying to be trauma informed for almost 15 years as I write this. In this time, I have studied, worked hard, reflected, tried, failed, learnt, and so on. But I wouldn't declare myself trauma informed, as it is an ongoing process that takes scrutiny, attention, and adaptation. Even if we know a lot about trauma, we cannot necessarily know what it takes to make everyone who has experienced trauma feel safe in our presence.

Nurses and midwives have always strived to deliver holistic care that adapts to the unique needs of the patient. Very few would ever strive to cause harm. Many nurses and midwives are trauma informed and have been, long before the phrase existed. However, if we say we are trauma informed without changing what we do, actively listening and engaging with people who have experienced care and found it harmful, or being open to the idea that everyone may not always find us to be safe and trustworthy, TIC becomes rhetoric. Using the language of TIC to describe care that isn't creates a disconnect between representation and reality which itself replicates harms. It can also become a form of 'epistemic gaslighting' (McKinnon, 2017). This is a misuse of power that directly contradicts what is to be trauma informed.

Yet we persist. For me, the persistence of TIC is linked to how I know it can change my own ways of being, while systems change is slower and requires solidarity and collective resistance. Often, I think about the reasons I stick with trauma informed care, despite the challenges it poses, despite the risks that it starts to sound like just being nice to everyone, and despite the deep conflicts that can arise in approaches to care, understandings of illness, and stressed healthcare systems. The reason for me is that in nursing situations of high intensity, emotion, and distress, and sometimes clinical stuckness, TIC has been one of the few things that has really made sense to me and that I've seen work. I've seen efforts towards TIC improve team morale and improve processes, environments, and structures of care. I've seen people who have worked for a very long time look at things differently when looking through a trauma lens, across all areas of health. I've seen dentists deliver intrusive procedures with safety and trust, emergency department staff respond differently to their most tricky customers, mental health services turn processes upside down to share power and create choice, and all parts of services working together to think differently about why people respond the way they do. And I've seen how, for me as a clinician, in slowing down and really asking myself what might have happened to this person in their life, what may be happening for this person right now, how might they be experiencing me, and what can I do in this moment to try to make them feel safer things can really shift. This is the trauma informed imagining. This is what reminds me of what is possible for trauma informed ways of being.

In healthcare, TIC requires two linked but separate processes that contribute to progress: consistent efforts towards preventing harm (including fear, shame, or retraumatisation), alosngside consistent efforts towards trauma sensitivity and responsiveness. Each of these is helpful, but both are needed. These can be targeted at individual practice, team processes, or organisational structures, and they should be adapted to different contexts, which means it is not possible for me or anyone to tell you what it looks like to be trauma informed. A key part of being trauma informed is attuning to the situation and adapting accordingly.

And, alongside this, there is a need for ongoing and sustained community outrage and activism against the perpetration of trauma, and also against the social structures that enable its ongoing harms. Being trauma informed in our practice will not solve systemic problems in healthcare, nor social issues that enable or support trauma. But it is an important concept to hold in mind when we engage closely with other humans during times of illness, pain, distress, or transformation. For me, being trauma informed is what has helped me stay in nursing, and what keeps me moving forward with it is that I see the power and possibility of it. I see what happens daily when people feel safe, or when staff are supported to do their work in ways that does not cause harm to them, or when links are made for people between how they feel in the present and what has happened to them in their lives. I have observed huge, profound shifts come from people understanding trauma in their lives. Being trauma informed also helps me to understand how to navigate tricky moments and how to be with people in ways that feel healing. I think we owe it to our patients to try to be trauma informed, but we also owe it to ourselves.

References

Burke-Harris, N. (Director). (2015). *How childhood trauma affects health across a lifetime* [Video recording]. https://www.ted.com/talks/nadine_burke_harris_how_childhood_trauma_affects_health_across_a_lifetime?language=en

Isobel, S., & Edwards, C. (2017). Using trauma informed care as a nursing model of care in an acute inpatient mental health unit: A practice development process. *International Journal of Mental Health Nursing, 26*(1), 88–94. https://doi.org/10.1111/inm.12236

McKinnon, R. (2017). Allies behaving badly: Gaslighting as epistemic injustice. In *The Routledge handbook of epistemic injustice* (pp. 167–174). Routledge.

Index

For Product Safety Concerns and Information please contact our EU
representative GPSR@taylorandfrancis.com
Taylor & Francis Verlag GmbH, Kaufingerstraße 24, 80331 München, Germany